Clinical Companion to Sleep Disorders Medicine
Second Edition

D0668750

Clinical Companion to Sleep Disorders Medicine
Second Edition

Sudhansu Chokroverty, M.D., F.R.C.P., F.A.C.P.

Professor of Neurology, New York Medical College, Valhalla; Clinical Professor of Neurology, University of Medicine and Dentistry of New Jersey—Robert Wood Johnson Medical School, Piscataway; Associate Chairman of Neurology, Chairman of Neurophysiology, and Director, Center of Sleep Medicine, Saint Vincents Hospital and Medical Center, New York

BUTTERWORTH
HEINEMANN

Boston   Oxford   Auckland   Johannesburg   Melbourne   New Delhi

MT

Library of Congress Cataloging-in-Publication Data
Chokroverty, Sudhansu.
  Clinical companion to Sleep disorders medicine Second edition / Sudhansu
  Chokroverty.
    p. ; cm.
  Companion v. to: Sleep disorders medicine / edited by Sudhansu Chokroverty.
  2nd ed. c1999.
  Includes bibliographical references and index.
  ISBN 0-7506-9687-7
   1. Sleep disorders. I. Title.
   [DNLM: 1. Sleep disorders. 2. Sleep--physiology. WM 188 C546c 2000]
  RC547 .C48 2000
  616.8'498--dc21
                                                                99-053900

British Library Cataloguing-in-Publication Data
A catalogue record for this book is available from the British Library.

The publisher offers special discounts on bulk orders of this book.

For information, please contact:
Manager of Special Sales
Butterworth–Heinemann
225 Wildwood Avenue
Woburn, MA 01801-2041
Tel: 781-904-2500
Fax: 781-904-2620

For information on all Butterworth–Heinemann publications available, contact our World Wide Web home page at: http://www.bh.com

10 9 8 7 6 5 4 3

Printed in the United States of America

2|1|06

Contents

Preface   *vii*

1. An Overview of Sleep   1

2. Neurophysiologic and Neurochemical Mechanisms
    of Wakefulness and Sleep   9

3. Physiologic Changes in Sleep   15

4. Polysomnography and Related Procedures   21

5. Measurement of Sleepiness and Alertness:
    Multiple Sleep Latency Test and Maintenance
    of Wakefulness Test   31

6. Sleep Scoring Technique   37

7. Classification and Approach to a Patient with
    Sleep Disorders   47

8. Epidemiology of Sleep Disorders   59

9. Genetics of Sleep and Sleep Disorders   65

10. Obstructive Sleep Apnea Syndrome   69

11. Insomnia   81

12. Narcolepsy and Idiopathic Hypersomnia   95

13. Motor Functions and Dysfunctions of Sleep   107

14. Sleep and Neurologic Disorders   127

15. Sleep in Psychiatric Disorders   145

16. Sleep Disturbances in Other Medical Disorders   151

17. Circadian Regulation of Sleep and Circadian
    Sleep Disorders   161

18. Parasomnias   167

19. Sleep Disorders in the Elderly   175

20.   Pediatric Sleep Disorders   187

21.   Sleep-Related Violence and Forensic Issues   193

Appendix: Glossary of Terms   199
Index   215

Preface

This companion handbook is a compressed version of the larger text, *Sleep Disorders Medicine: Basic Science, Technical Considerations, and Clinical Aspects*, Second Edition, published by Butterworth–Heinemann (1999). Several chapters from the original text, consisting of 35 chapters, have been condensed into a compact but comprehensive text of 21 chapters. This companion handbook addresses all of the elements necessary to practice sleep medicine. The text is augmented by including a number of tables for clarity and for a quick reference to the salient points. With the increasing awareness of the importance of a good night's sleep and the serious consequences resulting from sleep deprivation and sleep disorders, it is believed that a concise review in sleep medicine is needed for those physicians who are not sleep specialists. This companion handbook is not a substitute for the larger text, and readers are referred to the larger text for more in-depth and comprehensive coverage of sleep medicine.

Patients with sleep complaints often go to their primary care physicians, who are in the best position to diagnose sleep disorders and, if necessary, refer patients to sleep specialists. Therefore, it is incumbent on these physicians to have a broad general knowledge about sleep and its disorders. In addition to primary care physicians, internists, otolaryngologists, neurologists, psychiatrists, psychologists, pediatricians, geriatricians, residents, fellows, medical students, sleep technologists, and other individuals with an interest in sleep medicine should find this companion handbook useful.

I express my gratitude to Susan Pioli, Director of Medical Publishing, and Jodie Allen, Production Editor at Butterworth–Heinemann, as well as to the staff at Silverchair Science + Communications, without whose efforts this handbook would not have seen the daylight. I am also grateful to all the contributing authors for their scholarly contributions to the larger text, *Sleep Disorders Medicine: Basic Science, Technical Considerations, and Clinical Aspects*, Second Edition. I am indebted to my assistant Errika Thompson for typing and retyping all of the chapters in the companion handbook.

Last, but not least, I must express my appreciation to my wife, Manisha Chokroverty, M.D., for sacrificing all the precious summer weekends and even vacation time when I was busy compiling the companion handbook.

S. Chokroverty, M.D.

1

An Overview of Sleep

Human existence can be divided into three states: wakefulness, nonrapid eye movement (NREM) sleep, and rapid eye movement (REM) sleep. Sleep and wakefulness—the two basic processes of life—are like two different worlds with independent controls and functions. The fundamental questions of "What is sleep?" and "Why do we sleep?" have always baffled scientists. Poets, philosophers, writers, and religious scholars define sleep in their own ways, but a suitable scientific definition of sleep is lacking. The modern sleep scientist defines sleep on the bases of behavioral and physiologic criteria. Behavioral criteria (Table 1.1) include the following: lack of mobility or slight mobility, closed eyes, a characteristic sleepy posture, a markedly reduced response to external stimulation (e.g., increased arousal threshold), and a reversibly unconscious state. Physiologic criteria (Table 1.2) are based on the findings of electroencephalography (EEG), electro-oculography (EOG), and electromyography (EMG).

SLEEP ARCHITECTURE AND SLEEP STAGES

Based on physiologic criteria, sleep is divided into two independent states: NREM and REM sleep (Table 1.3). NREM sleep is further divided into four stages based primarily on EEG criteria. NREM and REM sleep alternate, with each cycle lasting approximately 90–110 minutes. Four to six such cycles are noted during normal sleep. The first third of normal sleep is dominated by slow wave sleep (SWS) (stages III and IV NREM sleep), and the last third is dominated by REM sleep. The first REM cycle is short; the last REM cycle (toward the end of the night or early hours of the morning) is generally the longest and can last up to an hour.

Nonrapid Eye Movement Sleep

NREM sleep accounts for 75–80% of sleep time in adult humans. Stage I NREM comprises 3–8% of sleep time; stage II occupies 45–55%; and stage III and IV make up 15–20% of total sleep time. In stage I NREM

Table 1.1
Behavioral criteria of wakefulness and sleep

Characteristics	Wakefulness	Nonrapid Eye Movement Sleep	Rapid Eye Movement Sleep
Posture	Erect, sitting, or recumbent	Recumbent	Recumbent
Mobility	Normal	Mildly reduced to absent; postural shifts	Moderately reduced to absent; myoclonic jerks
Response to stimulation	Normal	Mildly to moderately reduced	Moderately reduced to absent
Level of alertness	Alert	Unconscious but reversible	Unconscious but reversible
Eye position	Open	Closed	Closed
Eye movements	Waking eye movements	Slow eye movements	Rapid eye movements

Table 1.2
Physiologic criteria of wakefulness and sleep

Characteristics	Wakefulness	Nonrapid Eye Movement Sleep	Rapid Eye Movement Sleep
Electroencephalography	Parieto-occipital alpha waves (8–13 Hz) mixed with fronto-central beta rhythms (>13 Hz)	Theta (4–7 Hz) and delta (<4 Hz) waves, sleep spindles, vertex waves and K complexes	Theta or "saw tooth" waves, beta rhythms
Electromyography (muscle tone)	Normal	Mildly reduced	Markedly reduced to absent
Electrooculography	Waking eye movements	Slow eye movements	Rapid eye movements

sleep, the alpha rhythm (8–13 Hz), characteristic of wakefulness, diminishes to less than 50% in an epoch (i.e., a 30-second polysomnographic tracing with a speed of 10 mm per second), and a mixture of slower theta rhythms (4–7 Hz) and beta (greater than 13 Hz) waves appear. EMG activity decreases slightly and slow rolling eye movements may be

Table 1.3
Summary of nonrapid eye movement (NREM) and rapid eye movement (REM)
sleep stages

NREM sleep: 75–80% of sleep time
    Stage I: 3–8% of sleep time
    Stage II: 45–55% of sleep time
    Stage III: 3–8% of sleep time
    Stage IV: 10–15% of sleep time
REM sleep: 20–25% of sleep time
    Tonic stage
    Phasic stage

---

recorded. Vertex sharp waves are noted toward the end of stage I NREM
sleep. Stage II NREM sleep begins after approximately 10–12 minutes of
stage I NREM sleep. The characteristic EEG findings of stage II NREM
sleep include sleep spindles (12–18 Hz, most often 14 Hz) and K complexes intermixed with vertex sharp waves. Delta waves (less than 4 Hz)
in the EEG occupy less than 20% of the epoch. Stage II NREM sleep lasts
for approximately 30–60 minutes. During stage III NREM sleep, delta
waves occupy 20–50% of the epoch, and during stage IV NREM sleep,
delta waves occupy more than 50% of the epoch. Together, stages III and
IV NREM sleep constitute SWS. EOG does not register eye movements
in stages II to IV NREM sleep. Muscle tone, measured by EMG, is less
than in wakefulness or stage I sleep. Toward the end of SWS, body movements are registered as artifacts in polysomnographic recordings.

Rapid Eye Movement Sleep

REM sleep accounts for 20–25% of sleep time. The first REM sleep
episode is noted 60–90 minutes after the onset of NREM sleep. Based
on EEG, EMG, and EOG characteristics, REM sleep can be divided into
two stages, tonic and phasic. EEG tracings during REM sleep are characterized by fast rhythms and theta waves, some of which may have a
sawtooth appearance. Sawtooth waves are thought to be the gateway
to REM sleep. Characteristics of the tonic stage include desynchronized
EEG, hypotonia or atonia of major muscle groups, and depression of
monosynaptic and polysynaptic reflexes. Phasic REM sleep is characterized by rapid eye movements in all directions as well as by phasic
swings in blood pressure and heart rate, irregular respiration, spontaneous middle ear muscle activity, and tongue movements. A few periods of apnea or hypopnea may occur during REM sleep. Table 1.3
summarizes the characteristics of NREM and REM sleep stages.

EVOLUTION OF SLEEP PATTERNS
FROM INFANCY TO OLD AGE

Sleep requirements change dramatically from infancy to old age. New-borns have a polyphasic sleep pattern, sleeping approximately 16 hours per day. Sleep requirements fall to approximately 10 hours per day between ages 3 and 5 years. Preschool children assume biphasic sleep patterns, but adults exhibit a monophasic sleep pattern with an average duration of approximately 8 hours of sleep at night. This pattern becomes biphasic again in old age.

Newborn infants spend approximately 50% of sleep time in REM sleep, but by age 6 years, this time decreases to the normal adult pattern of 25%. After falling asleep, a newborn baby immediately goes into REM sleep, or active sleep, accompanied by restless movements of arms, legs, and facial muscles. (In premature babies, it is often difficult to differentiate REM sleep from wakefulness.) By age 3 months, the NREM–REM cyclic pattern of adult sleep is established; however, the NREM–REM cycle duration is shorter in infants, lasting approximately 45–50 minutes. Sleep cycle duration increases to 60–70 minutes between the ages of 5 and 10 years. By age 10 years, a normal adult cyclic pattern of 90–110 minutes is established. Sleep spindles begin to appear at approximately 3 months of age and K complexes are seen at approximately 6 months of age.

A characteristic feature of sleep in old age is marked attenuation of the amplitude of delta waves; therefore, during scoring of delta sleep, which depends not only on the frequency but also on the amplitude of delta, the percentage of delta decreases. Another notable feature of old age sleep patterns is repeated awakenings throughout the night and early morning. The percentage of REM sleep in normal elders remains relatively constant. Older people often complain of poor sleep quality caused by repeated awakenings. The total duration of sleep time within 24 hours in normal elderly people, however, is generally not different from that of young adults, because older individuals often nap during the daytime, compensating for lost sleep during the night.

CHRONOBIOLOGY AND CIRCADIAN RHYTHMS

The term *circadian rhythm* is derived from the Latin *circa*, which means "about," and *dien*, which means "day." The existence of circadian rhythms was first observed in 1731, when the French astronomer Jean Jacques Dortous de Mairan noted a circadian rhythm in a plant. The experimental isolation of humans from all environmental time cues, as in a cave or underground bunker (the German term *zeitgeber*) to study free-running rhythms, has demonstrated that circadian rhythms exist independent of environmental stimuli. The cycle lasts approximately 25 hours (range 24.7–25.2 hours) instead of 24 hours of day–night cycle. Normally, environmental cues of light and darkness synchronize or entrain rhythms to the day–night cycle; however, the existence of environment-independent autonomous rhythms suggests that the human body also has an internal biological clock. The site of this biological clock has been located in the paired suprachiasmatic nuclei of the hypothalamus above the optic chiasm. Time isolation experiments have shown that daily rhythms exist in many physiologic processes such as sleep, basic rest activity, body temperature, and neuroendocrine secretions. The most important of these rhythms is body temperature rhythm, which, although independent of the circadian rhythm of sleep/wakefulness, follows it closely. Dysfunction of circadian rhythms results in some important human sleep disorders (see Chapter 17).

SLEEP HABITS

Sleep specialists divide people into two groups depending on sleep habits: evening types and morning types. Evening types, or "owls," have difficulty getting up early and feel tired in the morning, but feel refreshed toward the end of the day. This group performs best in the evening and prefers to go to sleep late and wake up late. In contrast, morning types ("larks") wake up early, rested and refreshed, and work efficiently in the morning. Body temperature rhythms show two different curves for these two types of people, with an evening peak occurring 1 hour earlier in morning types than in evening types. Most likely, morning and evening types are determined by genetic factors.

SLEEP REQUIREMENTS

Average adults require approximately 8 hours of sleep, regardless of environmental or cultural differences. An important epidemiologic study found that the chances of death from coronary arterial disease, cancer, or stroke are greater for adults who sleep less than 4 hours or more than 9 hours as compared with those who sleep an average number of 8 hours. Most probably, whether a person is a "long" or "short" sleeper is determined by heredity rather than distinguished personality traits or other psychological factors. Long sleepers spend more time asleep but have fewer stage III and IV NREM sleep and more stage II NREM sleep than do short sleepers.

SLEEP AND DREAMS

Since the existence of REM sleep was first observed by Aserinksy and Kleitman in 1953, dream research has taken a new direction. It is now believed that approximately 80% of dreams occur during REM sleep and 20% occur during NREM sleep. REM sleep dreams appear to be highly emotionally charged, complex, and bizarre, whereas NREM dreams are more realistic and rational. On awakening from REM sleep, people are generally oriented; on awakening from NREM sleep, however, they are somewhat disoriented and confused. Although the significance of dreams remains unknown, some suggestions include activation of neural networks in the brain, restructuring and reinterpretation of data stored in memory, and removal of unnecessary and useless information from the brain.

CIRCADIAN, HOMEOSTATIC, AND OTHER SLEEP FACTORS

Sleep and wakefulness are controlled by homeostatic and circadian factors. Duration of prior wakefulness, the homeostatic factor, determines propensity to sleepiness, whereas the circadian factor determines timing, duration, and characteristics of sleep. There are two highly vulnerable periods of sleepiness: 3:00–5:00 AM and 3:00–5:00 PM; the former is stronger than the latter. The highest number of sleep-related accidents have been observed during these periods. Subjective sleepiness—an individual's perception of sleepiness—depends on several external factors, such as environment and ingestion of coffee or other caffeinated beverages. Physiologic sleepiness depends on homeostatic and circadian factors. The term *homeostatic factor* refers to a period of wakefulness and sleep debt. After a prolonged period of wakefulness, there is an increasing tendency to sleep. Recovery from sleep debt is aided by an additional amount of sleep, but this recovery is not linear. Thus, an exact number of hours of sleep are not required to repay sleep debt; rather, the body needs an adequate amount of SWS for restoration. Sleep–wakefulness and the circadian pacemaker have a reciprocal relationship, but the neurologic basis for this interaction is unknown.

The role of various sleep factors in maintaining homeostasis has not been clearly established. Several cytokines, including interleukin-1, interferon-α, and tumor necrosis factor, promote sleep. Other sleep-promoting substances, called *sleep factors*, increase in concentration during prolonged wakefulness or infection. Several endogenous compounds that are thought to enhance sleep have been identified: delta sleep—inducing peptides, muramyl peptides, cholecystokinins, arginine vasotocin, vasoactive intestinal peptide, growth hormone–releasing factors, and somatostatin. Adenosine may fulfill the major criteria for a neural sleep factor that mediates the somnogenic effects of prolonged wakefulness.

SLEEP DEPRIVATION AND SLEEPINESS

It is known that sleep is essential and a lack of sleep leads to sleepiness, but the exact functions of sleep are not known. Sleep deprivation experiments have proven that an impairment of human performance accompanies sleep deprivation, thus attesting to the need for sleep. Such experiments have shown that there is no permanent impairment of the human nervous system, but loss of performance does occur after long sleep deprivation as a result of decreased motivation and frequent microsleeps. Multiple sleep latency tests show that sleep deprivation increases tendency to sleep during daytime. It is also noted that the percentage of NREM stages III and IV or SWS increases considerably after sleep deprivation. REM sleep percentage also increases during recovery sleep after a long period of sleep deprivation. Minimal deficits in performance due to decreased motivation have been noted after partial sleep deprivation. Overall, sleep deprivation experiments have proved that sleep deprivation causes sleepiness and impairment of performance, vigilance, attention, and concentration, but does not cause permanent memory or other central nervous system changes.

FUNCTION OF SLEEP

Despite considerable progress in understanding the neurobiology of sleep, the exact biological function of sleep is still not known. Several theories of the function of sleep have been proposed (Table 1.4).

According to the restorative theory, NREM sleep is needed for body tissue restoration and REM sleep is needed for brain tissue restoration. Increased secretion of anabolic hormones (e.g., growth hormone, prolactin, testosterone, and luteinizing hormone), and decreased levels of catabolic hormone (e.g., cortisol) during sleep, as well as a subjective feeling of refreshment after sleep, may support the restorative theory. Increased SWS after sleep deprivation further suggests NREM sleep plays a role in restoring the body. Both the role of REM sleep in central nervous system development in young organisms and increased protein synthesis in the brain during REM sleep help support the theory that REM sleep restores brain function.

Table 1.4
Biological functions of sleep

Body and brain tissue restoration
Energy conservation
Adaptation
Memory reinforcement and consolidation
Synaptic and neural network integrity
Thermoregulation

Several studies of brain basal metabolism suggest an enhanced synthesis of macromolecules (such as nucleic acids and proteins) occurs in the brain during sleep, but data remain scarce and controversial.

The fact that animals with high metabolic rates sleep longer than those with slower metabolisms has been cited in support of energy conservation theory. It should be noted, however, that during 8 hours of sleep, only 120 calories are conserved.

Proponents of the adaptive theory suggest that sleep is an instinctual and adaptive behavior that allows creatures to survive under a variety of environmental conditions.

The theory of memory reinforcement and consolidation suggests that memory facilitation and learning take place during REM sleep. This theory has been strengthened by REM and SWS sleep deprivation experiments conducted in young adults, in whom perceptual learning during REM deprivation was significantly less than with SWS deprivation. These data suggest that REM deprivation affects the consolidation of recent perceptual experience.

The theory of maintenance of synaptic and neuronal network integrity is an emerging concept that is concerned with the primary function of sleep. Intermittent stimulation of neural network synapses is necessary to preserve CNS function. The concept of dynamic stabilization (repetitive activation of brain synapses and neural circuitry) suggests that REM sleep maintains motor circuits, whereas NREM sleep maintains nonmotor activities.

The theory of thermoregulatory function is based on the observation that thermoregulatory homeostasis is maintained during sleep, whereas severe thermoregulatory abnormalities follow total sleep deprivation. The influence of preoptic and anterior hypothalamic thermosensitive neurons on sleep and arousal can be cited as evidence for the thermoregulatory function of sleep.

2

Neurophysiologic and Neurochemical Mechanisms of Wakefulness and Sleep

The precise mechanisms of wakefulness, nonrapid eye movement (NREM) sleep and rapid eye movement (REM) sleep are not known, but a vast amount of information is available about neuroanatomic substrates, physiologic mechanisms based on the neuronal activity from unit recordings, and neurochemical substrates of these three states of human existence.

WAKEFULNESS AND AROUSAL

Two major systems are thought to be responsible for wakefulness, arousal, and cognition: the ascending reticular activating system (ARAS) in the upper brain stem, which sends projections to the posterior hypothalamus and forebrain regions, and the system responsible for cognition in the cerebral cortex and its subcortical connections. Marked impairment of the arousal and cognition systems may result in coma or severe sleepiness. The rapid reversibility of the state of awareness differentiates sleep from coma and death. Physiologic and metabolic differences between sleep and coma also exist. Coma is a passive process in which loss of function occurs, whereas sleep is an active state resulting from physiologic interactions of various systems in the brain stem and cerebral cortex. Also, metabolic depression of the cerebral cortex and brain stem characterizes coma and stupor, whereas in sleep, oxygen utilization and metabolism remain intact.

Projections from the ARAS, terminating in the thalamus and thalamocortical projections to widespread areas of the cerebral cortex, produce cerebral cortical activation during wakefulness. Extrathalamic projections from the brain stem reticular neurons terminate in the posterior hypothalamus and the basal forebrain regions; the latter, in turn, project to the cerebral cortex to maintain wakefulness. Wakefulness is a state of behavior characterized by alertness and readiness that is electrophysiologically manifested by electroencephalographic (EEG) evidence of parieto-occipital alpha waves and fronto-central fast waves in beta frequencies. Unit recordings of the ARAS and extrathalamic projections show high-frequency tonic firing rates during wakefulness.

The major neurotransmitter pathways that regulate the wakefulness systems (ARAS projecting to the thalamus, the hypothalamus, and basal forebrain) use the cholinergic, noradrenergic, dopaminergic, and histaminergic neurons. Cholinergic neurons in the laterodorsal and pedunculopontine tegmental nuclei at the pontomesencephalic junction project to the thalamus, posterior hypothalamus, and basal forebrain region (i.e., nucleus basalis of Meynert). These cholinergic neurons fire at their highest rates during wakefulness and during REM sleep but decrease their rates of firing at the onset of NREM sleep. Acetylcholine, through both nicotinic and muscarinic receptors, depolarizes and excites the thalamocortical projecting neurons, promoting tonic firing. Cholinergic receptor antagonists (e.g., scopolamine) inhibit cortical activation.

The role of dopamine is uncertain. However, pharmacologic, biochemical and physiologic studies suggest dopamine helps maintain wakefulness, probably through its D_1 (and possibly D_2) receptors.

Norepinephrine-containing locus ceruleus neurons show their highest firing rates during wakefulness, their lowest during REM sleep, and intermediate firing rates during NREM sleep. The noradrenergic system promotes wakefulness. The role of various noradrenergic receptor subtypes in maintaining sleep-wakefulness needs to be clarified.

Pharmacologic studies suggest posterior hypothalamic histaminergic neurons help maintain wakefulness and, possibly, vigilance.

The excitatory amino acids, glutamate and aspartate, are present in many neurons projecting to the cerebral cortex, forebrain and brain stem, and are released maximally during wakefulness. Glutamate or aspartate-containing neurons are intermingled within the ARAS. Prolonged cortical activation is produced by glutamate agonists.

Many peptides and hormones (corticotrophin-releasing factor, thyrotropin-releasing factor, vasoactive intestinal polypeptide, thyroid-stimulating hormone, epinephrine, and adrenocorticotrophic hormone) may participate in maintenance of wakefulness.

NONRAPID EYE MOVEMENT SLEEP

The neuroanatomic substrates for NREM and REM sleep are located in separate parts of the central nervous system (CNS). NREM/REM sleep cycling and generation depend on active and passive mechanisms. In the 1930s and 1940s, sleep physiologists emphasized passive sleep theory, but beginning in the late 1950s, emphasis was shifted toward active sleep mechanisms. Proponents of active and passive theories alike base their conclusions on stimulation, ablation, and lesion experiments. In the 1970s and 1980s, intracellular and extracellular recordings, combined with pharmacologic injections of chemicals into discrete areas, were used to support the various sleep mechanisms that most likely result from both passive and active processes. These two theories are complementary, not necessarily oppositional in nature. The most plausible theory is that sleep–wake states are produced by chains of interconnecting systems rather than by discrete centers.

Based on two classic preparations in cats, Bremer found that in *cerveau isolé* preparation (e.g., midcollicular transection), all specific sensory stimuli were withdrawn, and the animals were somnolent, whereas in *encéphale isolé* preparation (transection at C1 vertebral level to disconnect the entire brain from the spinal cord), such specific sensory stimuli maintained activation of the brain, and the animals were awake. In 1949, Moruzzi and Magoun postulated that withdrawal of nonspecific sensory stimuli of the ARAS is responsible for somnolence in *cerveau isolé* preparation. Wakefulness results from activation of the ARAS and diffuse thalamocortical projections. Subsequently, a midpontine pretrigeminal section in cats by Batini et al. produced EEG and behavioral signs of wakefulness, challenging passive theory. It was concluded that neurons in the brain located between the midcollicular and midpontine regions are responsible for wakefulness.

The active hypnogenic neurons responsible for NREM sleep are thought to be located primarily in the preoptic area of the anterior hypothalamus and basal forebrain area, based on findings from stimulation, lesion, and ablation studies, and extracellular and intracellular recordings. Electrical stimulation of the preoptic area, which produces EEG synchronization and behavioral state of sleep, supports the idea that active hypnogenic neurons in the preoptic area exist. Experiments in which insomnia resulted from lesions of the preoptic area also support the hypothesis that active hypnogenic neurons exist in the forebrain preoptic area. Insomnia caused by ibotenic lesions in the preoptic area also supports the active hypnogenic role of the preoptic area. In ibotenic lesion experiments, however, an injection of muscimol, a γ-aminobutyric acid (GABA) agonist, in the posterior hypothalamus transiently recovered sleep, suggesting that the sleep-promoting role of the anterior hypothalamus is dependent on the inhibition of posterior hypothalamic histaminergic-awakening neurons. Physiologic studies also showed that increased firing rates of basal forebrain neurons occur during the appropriate behavioral state.

In addition to the preoptic-anterior hypothalamic region, there is also evidence to indicate that the nucleus of the tractus solitarius (NTS) in the medulla is also involved in NREM sleep generation. An increase in the firing rate of neurons within the NTS during NREM sleep occurs, and low-frequency stimulation of the NTS also produces slow waves in the EEG, as noted during NREM sleep. NTS neurons are also reciprocally interconnected with cells in the midbrain EEG arousal region; during NREM sleep, there is active inhibition of the ARAS by the lower brain stem hypnogenic neurons.

Although the NTS may be considered a second NREM sleep regulatory region, the search for active hypnogenic neurons should be conducted in the region of the basal forebrain rather than in the region of the NTS, because the evidence is stronger for the preoptic than the NTS neurons.

Nonrapid Eye Movement Sleep Rhythms and Slow Cortical Oscillations

The following cells are responsible for NREM sleep oscillations: cortical pyramidal cells (PCs), reticulothalamic cells (REs), and thalamocortical (TC) neurons. PCs project to the thalamus, exciting both REs and TCs. Excitatory TC projections to the cortex also send collaterals to REs, which in turn send inhibitory projections to TCs, thus creating an interthalamic recurrent inhibitory circuit. Sleep spindles and delta and slow cortical waves are the three major sleep oscillators. Sleep spindles are generated by GABA-ergic RE cells, which generate rhythmic inhibitory postsynaptic potentials on TC cells. Delta waves are produced in both the cortex and thalamus. During NREM sleep, hyperpolarization of TC cells results from withdrawal of activation of ARAS. At the onset of NREM sleep, deafferentation of the brain occurs, owing to initial blockage of afferent information at the thalamic level, causing the waking open brain to be converted into a closed brain as a result of thalamocortical inhibition.

Slow cortical oscillations of less than 1 Hz (typically 0.6–0.9 Hz) are generated within the cortical cells as a result of prolonged depolarization and hyperpolarization. K complex is considered the depth-negative slow oscillation. Slow oscillations are prominent in the frontoparietal region; their major component is hyperpolarization in the thalamic or cortical neurons. These oscillations disconnect the brain from the external world. Slow oscillations may play a role in plasticity and memory.

Several humoral sleep factors have been postulated to promote NREM sleep, including prostaglandin D_2, growth hormone–releasing factor, muramyl peptides, interleukins, and cholecystokinin. The role of these postulated humoral sleep factors, however, remains undetermined in the absence of experiments designed to test them at the cellular level in critical brain areas. It has been suggested that adenosine, a neuromodulator, may act as a physiologic sleep factor that modulates the somnogenic effects of prolonged wakefulness. This suggestion was postulated after experiments in cats showed that adenosine extracellular concentration in the basal forebrain cholinergic region increased progressively during prolonged spontaneous wakefulness.

Serotonin, located in the midline raphe neurons, was at one time thought to play an active role in the generation of NREM sleep. Many subsequent results, however, contradicted the original conclusion. The serotonergic dorsal raphe neurons projecting diffusely to the forebrain show their highest firing pattern during wakefulness, decrease their firing rate during NREM sleep, and are silent during REM sleep. GABA, an inhibitory neurotransmitter, is located within many neurons in the brain stem, thalamus, hypothalamus, basal forebrain, and cerebral cortex. GABA is thought to play a role in NREM sleep and is released maximally during NREM sleep. Benzodiazepines and barbiturates, which produce sedation, act on GABA receptors. GABA may be an important factor in suppressing the firing of neurons within the reticular activating system.

RAPID EYE MOVEMENT SLEEP

Jouvet's experiments in cats clearly documented that REM sleep–generating neurons are located in pons. A transection at the junction of pons and midbrain produced all of the physiologic findings compatible with REM sleep in the section caudal to the transection, whereas in the forebrain region rostral to the section, recordings showed no signs of REM sleep. After a transection between the pons and medulla, structures rostral to the section showed signs of REM sleep, but in structures caudal to the section, there were no signs of REM sleep. Also, after a section at the junction of the spinal cord and medulla, REM sleep signs were noted in the rostral brain areas. Finally, transection at the pontomesencephalic and at the pontomedullary junctions produced an isolated pons that showed all the signs of REM sleep. Therefore, from these experiments, it was concluded that pons is sufficient and necessary to generate all the signs of REM sleep.

Neurons in the pedunculopontine tegmental (PPT) nucleus and the laterodorsal tegmental (LDT) nucleus in the pontomesencephalic region are cholinergic; they are the REM-on cells, which are responsible for REM sleep and show high firing rates at this stage. The REM-off cells are located in the locus ceruleus and raphe nucleus; these cells are aminergic neurons and are quite inactive during REM sleep. Thus, the cholinergic REM-on and the aminergic REM-off neurons are all located between transections in the pons. A reciprocal interaction between REM-on and REM-off neurons in the brain stem are responsible for REM generation and maintenance. Pharmacologic and neurophysiologic evidence suggests that aminergic cells play a permissive role in the appearance of the REM sleep state. Cholinergic neurons of PPT and LDT project to the thalamus and basal forebrain regions, as well as to the medial pontine reticular formation. These neurons are responsible for activation and generation of REM sleep. Histamine-containing neurons are other REM-off neurons located in the posterior hypothalamus. These are wakefulness-promoting neurons and are not needed for REM sleep oscillations.

Muscle hypotonia or atonia during REM sleep is thought to depend on inhibitory postsynaptic potentials generated by dorsal pontine–descending axons. The pathway from the perilocus ceruleus alpha region ventral to the locus ceruleus via the lateral tegmentoreticular tract to the medial medullary region (e.g., nucleus magnocellularis and paramedianus) and then to the reticulospinal tract, projecting to the spinal cord's anterior horn cells, controls REM sleep–induced muscle atonia. An experimental lesion in the perilocus ceruleus alpha region produced REM sleep without muscle atonia.

3

Physiologic Changes in Sleep

A variety of physiologic changes occur during nonrapid eye movement (NREM) and rapid eye movement (REM) sleep that are different from those noted during wakefulness (Table 3.1). These changes are most commonly observed in the somatic and autonomic nervous systems; they include changes in the respiratory, cardiovascular, and gastrointestinal systems; endocrine, renal, and sexual functions; and thermoregulation. An understanding of physiologic changes in several body systems is important to understand the pathophysiology of many medical disorders, including disturbances of sleep.

SOMATIC CENTRAL NERVOUS SYSTEM

Firing rates of many neurons in the central nervous system (CNS) decrease during NREM sleep but increase during REM sleep.

AUTONOMIC NERVOUS SYSTEM

During sleep, there are profound changes in the functions of the autonomic nervous system (ANS) (Table 3.2). During NREM sleep, an overall tonic increase in parasympathetic activity occurs; it increases further during tonic REM sleep. Additionally, during phasic REM sleep, sympathetic activity decreases. However, sympathetic activity during REM sleep increases intermittently, resulting in swings of blood pressure and heart rate, causing bradytachyarrhythmias. Most autonomic changes involve the heart, circulation, respiration, thermoregulation, and pupils.

Table 3.1
Summary of physiologic changes during wakefulness, nonrapid eye movement (NREM) sleep, and rapid eye movement (REM) sleep

Physiologic	Wakefulness	NREM Sleep	REM Sleep
Parasympathetic activity	++	+++	++++
Sympathetic activity	++	+	± or variable (++)
Heart rate	Normal sinus rhythm	Bradycardia	Bradytachy-arrhythmia
Blood pressure	Normal	Decreases	Variable
Cardiac output	Normal	Decreases	Decreases further
Peripheral vascular resistance	Normal	Normal or decreases slightly	Decreases further
Respiratory rate	Normal	Decreases	Variable; apneas may occur
Alveolar ventilation	Normal	Decreases	Decreases further
Upper airway muscle tone	++	+	± or −
Upper airway resistance	++	+++	++++
Hypoxic ventilatory response	Normal	Decreases	Decreases further
Hypercapnic ventilatory response	Normal	Decreases	Decreases further
Cerebral blood flow	++	++ or +	++++

± = Minimal to absent; + = minimal; ++ = mild; +++ = moderate; ++++ = marked; − = absent.

Pupillary Changes

Pupilloconstriction occurs during NREM sleep and is maintained during REM sleep, owing to tonic parasympathetic drive. Pupillodilatation during phasic REM sleep results from a central inhibition of parasympathetic outflow to the iris.

Sympathetic Activity in Muscle and Skin Blood Vessels

The microneurographic technique, which measures sympathetic activity in muscle and skin vascular beds, reveals a reduction in muscles' sympathetic nerve activity during NREM sleep but an increment to levels above waking values during REM sleep, particularly during phasic REM sleep (see Table 3.2). In addition, there are transient bursts of sympathetic activity during arousal in NREM sleep.

Table 3.2
Autonomic nervous system changes during sleep

Nonrapid eye movement sleep
   Increased parasympathetic activity
   Decreased sympathetic activity
Rapid eye movement sleep
   More marked increase in parasympathetic activity
   Further decrease in sympathetic activity
   Intermittent increase in sympathetic activity in phasic rapid eye
      movement sleep
   Profound increase in sympathetic activity in skin and muscle vessels
      (according to microneurographic recordings)

RESPIRATION AND SLEEP

Two systems—metabolic, or automatic, and voluntary, or behavioral—control respiration during sleep and wakefulness. Both metabolic and voluntary systems operate during wakefulness, whereas only the metabolic system operates during NREM sleep. The wakefulness stimulus, probably derived from the ascending reticular activating system, represents a tonic stimulus to ventilation during wakefulness. During both NREM and REM sleep, respiratory neurons in the pontomedullary regions show decreased firing rates. Muscle tone in the upper airway decreases slightly in NREM sleep—but decreases markedly during REM sleep—resulting in an increase in upper airway resistance.

Decreased sensitivity of respiratory neurons to carbon dioxide, inhibition of the reticular activating system, and alteration of metabolic control of respiratory neurons during sleep result in a decrement of tidal volume and minute and alveolar ventilation. Diminished alveolar ventilation in normal individuals causes a mild decrement of arterial oxygen tension and a mild increment of arterial carbon dioxide tension. Oxygen saturation decreases by less than 2% during sleep. These changes occur despite a decrease in oxygen consumption and carbon dioxide production during sleep.

Hypercapnic and hypoxic ventilatory responses decrease during REM and NREM sleep, with more marked decreases during REM sleep. Arousal responses also decrease, particularly during REM sleep.

Respiration is, therefore, vulnerable during normal sleep, and a few periods of apneas may occur, especially at the onset of sleep and during REM sleep.

CHANGES IN THE CARDIOVASCULAR SYSTEM DURING SLEEP

Heart rate, systemic blood pressure, cardiac output, and peripheral vascular resistance decrease during NREM sleep; they decrease further during REM sleep. During phasic REM sleep, blood pressure and heart rate become unstable, due to phasic vagal inhibition and sympathetic activation caused by alterations in brain stem neural activity. Heart rate and blood pressure fluctuate during REM sleep; pulmonary arterial pressure, in contrast, rises slightly during NREM and REM sleep.

Cerebral blood flow and cerebral metabolic glucose and oxygen rates decrease during NREM sleep, whereas these values increase above those of waking levels during REM sleep. These data indirectly suggest that NREM sleep is the state of the resting brain, with reduced neuronal activity, decreased synaptic transmission, and depressed cerebral metabolism. The data also are consistent with the assumption that REM sleep represents an active brain state with increased neuronal activity and brain metabolism. The largest increase during REM sleep occurs in the hypothalamus and brain stem structures, and the smallest increases occur in the cerebral cortex and white matter.

CHANGES IN THE ALIMENTARY SYSTEM DURING SLEEP

Swallowing is suppressed during sleep, resulting in prolonged mucosal contact with refluxed acid. Salivary flow, important for acid neutralization, also is decreased during sleep, a phenomenon that contributes to prolonged acid clearance. Esophageal motility is reduced during sleep. All of these factors affect the pathogenesis of esophagitis caused by nocturnal gastroesophageal reflux.

Gastric acid secretion shows a variable response during sleep in normal individuals, but patients with duodenal ulcers show striking increases in acid secretion with no inhibition of secretion during the first 2 hours of sleep. Studies of intestinal motility during sleep are contradictory. A special pattern of motor activity, called *migrating motor complex*, shows a circadian rhythm in its propagation, with the slowest velocity during sleep. Thus, sleep-related changes in the enteric nervous system, a component of ANS, cause decreases in motor and secretory functions of the alimentary system.

CHANGES IN ENDOCRINE FUNCTION
DURING SLEEP

Profound changes in neuroendocrine secretions occur during sleep. Growth hormone secretion exhibits a pulsatile increase in NREM sleep during the first one-third of the night. Prolactin secretion also rises 60–90 minutes after the onset of sleep. Testosterone levels in adult men continue to be at their highest point during sleep, but no clear relation has been demonstrated between levels of gonadotropic hormones and the sleep–wake cycle in children or adults. During puberty, gonadotropin levels during sleep increase.

Secretion of thyroid-stimulating hormone reaches a peak in the evening and then decreases throughout the night. Sleep inhibits cortisol secretion. Melatonin, which is synthesized and released by the pineal gland and derived from serotonin, begins to rise in the evening, reaching its maximal values between 3:00 AM and 5:00 AM and decreasing to low levels during the day.

Other endocrine changes include a maximum rise in aldosterone just before awakening in the early hours of the morning and a marked decrease of plasma renin activity during REM sleep. Antidiuretic hormone shows episode secretion without any relationship to sleep or sleep stages. In persons with normal endocrine function, nocturnal urine volume decreases with decrement of glomerular filtration, alteration of renin release, and increased reabsorption of water.

CHANGES IN SEXUAL FUNCTION DURING SLEEP

The most striking finding is increased penile tumescence in men during REM sleep. In women, there is increased clitoral tumescence during REM sleep.

CHANGES IN THERMOREGULATION
DURING SLEEP

Body temperature is linked intimately to the sleep–wake cycle, but it follows a circadian rhythm independent of sleep–wake rhythm. At the onset of sleep, body temperature begins to fall; it reaches its lowest point during the third sleep cycle. Thermoregulation is maintained during NREM sleep but is nonexistent in REM sleep, and experimental animals have become poikilothermic; thus, physiologic responses to thermal stimuli (e.g., shivering, panting, sweating, and piloerection) are either depressed or absent during REM sleep.

CLINICAL IMPLICATIONS OF PHYSIOLOGIC CHANGES IN SLEEP

Multiple system atrophy, familial dysautonomia, and other conditions causing secondary autonomic failure adversely affect respiratory and cardiovascular functions during sleep, causing sleep-related respiratory dysrhythmias or even cardiac arrhythmias. Profound hemodynamic changes (e.g., unstable blood pressure and heart rate, and progressive decrease in cardiac output causing maximum oxygen desaturation and periodic breathing) and sympathetic alterations, which decrease with intermittent increase during REM sleep, may explain increasing mortality during early morning hours, especially in patients with cardiopulmonary disease. These hemodynamic and sympathetic alterations may initiate increased platelet aggregation, plaque rupture, and coronary arterial spasm, which may trigger thrombotic events that cause myocardial infarction, ventricular arrhythmia, and even sudden cardiac death and stroke.

Sleep-related alveolar hypoventilation and increased upper airway resistance may predispose susceptible individuals to upper airway occlusion and obstructive apnea. Patients with neuromuscular disorders, chronic obstructive pulmonary disease, and bronchial asthma may be affected adversely by such hypoventilation. Asthmatic attacks may be exacerbated at night as a result of bronchoconstriction during sleep.

Disruption of the linkage of thermoregulation and slow wave sleep, causing difficulty in initiating and maintaining sleep, and disruption of sleep architecture and daytime function, occur in subjects with jet lag and in shift workers. Menopausal hot flashes are thought to be a disorder of thermoregulation that initiates within preoptic-anterior hypothalamic neurons. The central thermoregulatory mechanisms underlying hot flashes may affect hypnogenic pathways, inducing sleep and causing heat loss in these patients. It is also suggested that thermoregulatory dysfunction may cause sleep disturbance in patients with depression, but there is no compelling evidence to support such an assumption.

Finally, disruption of the link between growth hormone secretion and slow wave sleep may cause sleep disturbance in patients with narcolepsy, sleep apnea, Cushing's syndrome, thyrotoxicosis, alcoholism, and in some cases of insomnia, as well as in elderly subjects. Melatonin secretion at night was found to be subnormal in a subgroup of elderly insomniacs; melatonin was administered to treat sleep disturbances in this subgroup, with beneficial effect.

4

Polysomnography and Related Procedures

Polysomnographic (PSG) study is the single most important laboratory technique used in the diagnosis and treatment of sleep disorders, especially those associated with excessive daytime somnolence. The term *PSG* was proposed in 1974 to describe the technique of recording, analyzing, and interpreting multiple simultaneous physiologic characteristics during sleep. An all-night PSG is required instead of a single nap study because a single nap study generally bypasses rapid eye movement (REM) sleep, the stage in which most severe apneic episodes are noted. Maximum oxygen desaturation also occurs at this stage; therefore, a daytime study cannot assess the severity of symptoms. Furthermore, during continuous positive airway pressure (CPAP) titration, an all-night sleep study is essential to determine the optimal level of pressure; therefore, both REM and nonrapid eye movement (NREM) sleep are required. An adequate clinical assessment of the patient is a prerequisite to PSG study. In this section, a brief review of the PSG technique and indications are briefly outlined.

PATIENT PREPARATION AND LABORATORY ENVIRONMENT

The technologist performing the study must have full clinical information so that he or she may make the necessary protocol adjustments for the most efficient recording. On arrival, the patient should be shown through the laboratory and adequately informed about the entire procedure. The laboratory should be located in an area that is free from noise, and the room should be kept at an optimal temperature. The idea is to provide a comfortable room, similar to the patient's bedroom at home, so that it is easy for the patient to relax and fall asleep. The recording equipment should be in an adjacent room. The patient should be advised about audiovisual equipment. A pre- and poststudy sleep questionnaire helps determine the patient's perception of the quality of his or her sleep and the actual test results.

TECHNICAL CONSIDERATIONS

PSG includes simultaneous recording of various physiologic characteristics, which allows assessment of sleep stages and wakefulness, respiration, cardiocirculatory functions, and body movements. Sleep staging is based on electroencephalogram (EEG), electro-oculogram (EOG), and electromyogram (EMG) of some skeletal muscles, especially chin muscles. PSG study also records airflow, respiratory effort, electrocardiogram (ECG), oxymetry, and limb muscle activity (particularly EMG of the tibialis anterior muscles bilaterally). It is advantageous to record snoring and body positions. Some laboratories also record intraesophageal pressure and esophageal pH.

It is important to calibrate the equipment to ensure adequate function of amplifiers and that settings are appropriate for the particular protocol. After the application of electrodes and other monitors, physiologic calibration is performed to document their proper functioning. Table 4.1 lists the instructions given for physiologic calibrations.

It is important to understand the low- and high- frequency filters and sensitivity for the purpose of recording various physiologic characteristics optimally. For recording EEG, EOG, EMG, and ECG, differential alternating current (AC) amplifiers are used. These amplifiers can also be used to record airflow and breathing effort. Direct current (DC) amplifiers with no low-frequency filters are used to record slower

Table 4.1
Instructions for physiologic calibrations

Open eyes and look straight for 30 secs
Close eyes for 30 secs
Look left, right, up, and down
Blink eyes five times
Clench teeth
Inhale and exhale
Hold breath for 10 secs
Extend right hand and then left hand
Dorsiflex right foot and then left foot

Table 4.2
Filter and sensitivity settings for polysomnographic studies

Characteristics	High-Frequency Filter (Hz)	Time Constant (sec)	Low-Frequency Filter (Hz)	Sensitivity
Electroencephalogram	70 or 35	0.4	0.3	5–7 µV/mm
Electro-oculogram	70 or 35	0.4	0.3	5–7 µV/mm
Electromyogram	90	0.04	5.0	2–3 µV/mm
Electrocardiogram	15	0.12	1.0	1 mV/cm to start; adjust
Airflow and effort	15	1	0.1	5–7 µV/mm; adjust

moving potentials, such as oximeter or pH meter output, pressure during CPAP titration, and intraesophageal pressure changes or body positions. Table 4.2 lists filter settings and sensitivities.

The standard speed for recording traditional PSG is 10 mm per second so that each monitor screen or page is a 30-second epoch. In patients with suspected nocturnal seizures, however, a 30-mm-per-second recording speed is used for easy identification of epileptiform spike activities.

Digital system recordings are being used increasingly in laboratories. The advantages of digital recordings include greater flexibility in manipulating filter settings, sensitivity, and in reformatting montages after data collection. The other great advantage of computer-assisted recording includes storage and manipulation of data after collection. It is, however, recommended that adequate digital-to-analog conversion is available to produce a high-quality paper output.

ELECTROENCEPHALOGRAPHY

According to Rechtschaffen and Kales' technique for sleep staging, standard electrode derivations are C3/A2 or C4/A1. The amplitude criteria for sleep scoring applies to these derivations only. To score stage I sleep accurately, however, it is advantageous to include occipital electrodes (O1, O2) to identify alpha activity and its disappearance. Multiple EEG channels of recordings are preferable to one or two channels for documenting focal and diffuse neurologic lesions, accurately localizing epileptiform discharges in patients with seizure disorders, and

Table 4.3
Typical overnight polysomnographic montage with continuous positive airway pressure titration used in our laboratory*

Channel Number	Name
1	F3-C3
2	F7-T3
3	T3-T5
4	T5-O1
5	F4-C4
6	F8-T4
7	T4-T6
8	T6-O2
9	C3-A2
10	C4-A1
11	Left electro-oculogram
12	Right electro-oculogram
13	Chin electromyogram (EMG)
14	Left tibialis EMG
15	Right tibialis EMG
16	Oronasal
17	Chest
18	Abdomen
19	Snoring
20	Electrocardiogram
21	Heart rate
22	Position
23	Arterial oxygen saturation
24	Continuous positive airway pressure

*Channels 1–10 record electroencephalogram using the 10-20 International System of electrode placement. Channel 16 records airflow. Channels 17 and 18 record respiratory effort.

more accurately determining various sleep stages, awakenings, and transient events such as arousals.

A gold cup electrode with a hole in the center or silver–silver chloride electrodes are commonly used to record EEG. The 10-20 International System of electrode placement is the accepted standard for electrode placement and designing montages. Electrode impedance must be less than 5,000 Ω. Table 4.3 lists the EEG montages and other monitors we used to record an all-night PSG study in our laboratory.

ELECTRO-OCULOGRAPHY

EOG records corneoretinal (a relative positivity at the cornea and a relative negativity at the retina) potential difference. Any movement of the eyes changes the orientation of the dipole. A typical electrode (gold cup or silver–silver chloride) placement is 1 cm superior and lateral to the outer canthus of one eye with a second electrode placed 1 cm inferior and lateral to the outer canthus of the opposite eye. Both of these electrodes are then connected to a single reference electrode, either the same ear or the mastoid process of the temporal bone. In this arrangement, conjugate eye movements produce out-of-phase deflections in the two channels, whereas the EEG slow activity contaminating the eye electrodes is in-phase.

ELECTROMYOGRAPHY

Mental or submental EMG activity is monitored to record axial muscle tone, which is significantly decreased during REM sleep. In patients with bruxism (tooth grinding), an additional electrode may be placed over the masseter muscle.

In a standard PSG recording, EMGs are also recorded from the right and left tibialis anterior muscles to detect periodic limb movements in sleep (PLMS). In patients with suspected REM sleep behavior disorder, it is advantageous to place additional electrodes in the upper limbs (e.g., extensor digitorum communis muscles), because in some patients, muscle bursts during REM sleep are seen only in the upper extremities rather than in leg muscles. Multiple muscle EMG recordings that include all four limbs are important in patients with nocturnal paroxysmal dystonia, which is thought to be a form of frontal lobe seizure. In this condition, patients display dystonic-choreoathetoid movements; surface EMGs, in addition to video recordings, are necessary to record these activities.

ELECTROCARDIOGRAPHY

A single channel of ECG is sufficient for PSG recording; place one electrode over the sternum and the other electrode at a lateral chest location. This recording detects bradytachyarrhythmias or other arrhythmias seen in patients with obstructive sleep apnea syndrome (OSAS).

RESPIRATORY MONITORING DURING SLEEP

It is important to monitor respiration during PSG for the detection of apnea, hypopneas, and other respiratory dysrhythmias. To characterize breathing disturbance, we record air exchange (airflow) through the mouth and nose, as well as the respiratory effort that monitors respiratory muscle activity (manifested by expansion and relaxation of the thorax and abdomen) in our laboratory. Semiquantitative indirect methods are most commonly used.

A thermistor or a thermocouple device between the nose and mouth is commonly used to monitor airflow to detect changes in temperature (e.g., cool air during inspiration and warm air during expiration). A thermistor consisting of wires registers changes in electrical resistance, and thermocouples consisting of dissimilar metals (e.g., copper and constantin) register changes in voltage that result from temperature variations.

Devices used to record respiratory effort include mercury strain gauges, intercostal EMG, magnetometers, inductive plethysmography, and, more commonly, piezoelectric strain gauges, which permit differentiation between abdominal and thoracic movements. Piezoelectric strain gauges consist of a crystal that emits an electrical signal in response to pressure. For all of these devices, except intercostal EMG, one belt is placed around the chest and another one is placed around the abdomen, which allows detection of the paradoxical movements indicative of upper airway OSAS.

OXYGEN SATURATION

Finger pulse oximetry is routinely used to monitor arterial oxygen saturation (Sao_2), or arterial oxyhemoglobin saturation, which reflects the percentage of hemoglobin that is oxygenated. The difference in light absorption between oxyhemoglobin and deoxyhemoglobin determines oxygen saturation. Continuous monitoring of Sao_2 is crucial because it provides important information about the severity of respiratory dysfunction.

EXPIRED CARBON DIOXIDE

Capnography detects the expired carbon dioxide (CO_2) level, which closely approximates intra-alveolar CO_2. Thus, capnography detects both airflow and the partial pressure of CO_2 in alveoli, which is useful for evaluating OSAS or other underlying pulmonary disease. Capnography is more sensitive than thermocouples or thermistors, but it is much more costly and, therefore, is not used in most laboratories.

INTRAESOPHAGEAL PRESSURE MONITORING

Intraesophageal pressure monitoring is a sensitive technique for measuring respiratory effort. It is, however, an invasive method, and requires placing a nasogastric balloon-tipped catheter into the distal esophagus. It is also the only way to detect with certainty the presence of upper airway resistance syndrome and is sometimes useful in distinguishing central from obstructive apnea.

OTHER MONITORING METHODS

Snoring

Snoring can be monitored by placing a miniature microphone on the patient's neck.

Esophageal pH

Esophageal pH is monitored by asking patients to swallow a pH probe. Recording the output using a DC amplifier may be useful in detecting nocturnal gastroesophageal reflux. Reflux disease may be mistaken for sleep apnea or nocturnal angina, as the patient may wake up choking or have severe chest pain as a result of acid eructation.

Video Monitoring

Video monitoring patient behavior during sleep is important in diagnosing parasomnias or nocturnal seizures. Monitoring also detects the abnormal shakes and jerks noted in patients with upper airway OSAS syndrome. A closed circuit television with online display in the monitor allows a detailed review of any abnormal events.

Body Position

Body position is monitored by placing sensors over one shoulder and using a DC channel. Snoring and apneas are generally worse in the supine position, and, therefore, CPAP titration must include observing patients in the supine position for evaluating optimal pressure for titration.

A typical montage used in our laboratory is shown in Table 4.3.

MONITORING AND RECORDING

Complete documentation, including the patient's name and record number, date of recording, description of study, name of technologist, and name(s) of equipment used, is essential. Beginning recording time is noted by "lights out," and ending time is indicated by "lights on." The technologist also should provide a clinical description of any unusual events that occur. Ideally, the patient should be recorded for 8 hours. When the patient is awoken, physiologic and biological calibrations should be performed. The patient is asked to fill out a post-study questionnaire, which includes his or her estimation of time required to fall asleep, total amount of time spent in sleep, awakenings, and quality of sleep.

INDICATIONS FOR POLYSOMNOGRAPHY

The American Sleep Disorders Association (ASDA), now known as the American Academy of Sleep Medicine, has proposed the following guidelines for indicating overnight polysomnography:

1. PSG is routinely indicated for the diagnosis of sleep-related breathing disorders.
2. PSG is indicated for CPAP titration in patients with sleep-related breathing disorders.
3. PSG is indicated to evaluate the presence of OSAS in patients before they undergo laser-assisted uvulopalatopharyngoplasty.
4. PSG is indicated for assessing therapeutic benefits after dental appliance treatment or after surgical treatment with moderately severe OSAS, including for those patients whose symptoms reappear despite an initial good response.
5. A follow-up PSG is indicated for assessment of treatment if the patient has lost or gained substantial weight, when the clinical response is insufficient, or when symptoms return despite a good initial response to treatment with CPAP.
6. For the diagnosis of suspected narcolepsy, an overnight PSG followed by multiple sleep latency tests are routinely indicated.
7. PSG is indicated in patients with parasomnias that are unusual or atypical, or if behaviors are violent or otherwise injurious to the

patient or others. PSG, however, is not routinely indicated in uncomplicated and typical parasomnias.

8. PSG is indicated in patients suspected of nocturnal seizures.
9. Overnight PSG is required in patients with suspected PLMS, but it is not performed routinely to diagnose restless legs syndrome.
10. PSG may be indicated for patients with insomnia who have not responded satisfactorily to a comprehensive behavioral or pharmacologic treatment program for the management of insomnia. In patients with insomnia, however, if there is a strong suspicion that sleep-related breathing disorder or associated PLMS is present, PSG study is indicated.

PORTABLE SLEEP RECORDING

Standard polysomnographic recording attended continuously by an experienced technologist in a laboratory is the standard in PSG recording for diagnosing OSAS and other sleep disorders. Because overnight PSG studies in laboratories are labor-intensive and expensive, there has been a rapid increase in the use of portable recordings to perform more quick and convenient tests at reduced costs. Portable recording is unattended; therefore, although it is cheaper, it is not necessarily a better method of evaluation. The advantages of portable recording include easy accessibility, convenience, patient acceptability and familiarity with sleep environment, and reduced operating costs. However, there are serious limitations of unattended portable recordings. In unattended recordings, a trained technologist is not available to correct any artifacts that may arise during recording or make appropriate equipment adjustments, and there is an absence of behavioral correlation with the recordings. For CPAP titration, an in-house attended recording is required. In the future, however, with the refinement and validity of automated CPAP titration, and with proper refinement of recording equipment, portable unattended recordings may be performed more often.

The ASDA standards of practice list the following guidelines. Portable studies are indicated.

- For patients with severe clinical symptoms indicative of a diagnosis of OSAS when a standard PSG is not readily available.
- For patients unable to be studied in a sleep laboratory because they are nonambulatory and medically unstable and cannot be readily or safely moved to another location.
- For follow-up studies when a diagnosis has been made with standard PSG and therapy has been initiated. The intent is to evaluate response to therapy.

The ASDA also specifies that if portable studies are indicated, only level II and III studies are acceptable for diagnosis and assessment of therapy for patients with OSAS. Body positions must also be documented during recording to assess the presence of OSAS, and the raw data must be stored and readily available for review.

Other recommendations of the ASDA include the ordering of the request by a licensed physician, performance of the test by a trained technologist, and interpretation by a physician who is fully trained in sleep medicine.

Prospective and long-term studies comparing portable recording with in-house laboratory recording should be performed before routinely recommending portable PSG recording.

5

Measurement of Sleepiness and Alertness: Multiple Sleep Latency Test and Maintenance of Wakefulness Test

MULTIPLE SLEEP LATENCY TEST

Excessive daytime somnolence (EDS) is a major symptom of many sleep disorders and a public health problem. Its basic neural mechanism, however, is not known. Obtaining the history and performing a physical examination are the two most important initial steps in assessing subjects with EDS. Clinical assessment should be directed at diagnosing the presence of excessive sleepiness and at uncovering the causes of EDS. The following features suggest the presence of excessive sleepiness: subject falls asleep in inappropriate places and under inappropriate circumstances (e.g., subject sleeps while sitting down, watching television, reading, watching movies, sitting in classes or conferences, listening to a lecture, or, in severe cases, talking on the telephone); subject dozes off during routine tasks such as driving; subject complains of poor attention span and finds it difficult to cope at work and school or may be involved in accidents at work; sleep is nonrefreshing in quality; and subject takes frequent naps (often more than once a day).

A variety of scales have been developed to assess subjective degrees of sleepiness. The Stanford Sleepiness Scale (Table 5.1) is a seven-point scale used to measure subjective sleepiness; however, it may not be reliable in patients with persistent sleepiness. Another scale used to assess sleepiness is the Visual Analog Scale of Alertness and Well-Being, in which subjects indicate their feelings and alertness at an arbitrary point on a line. This scale has been used successfully in treating circadian rhythm disorders. The Epworth Sleepiness Scale evaluates general levels of sleepiness. In it, the patients rate eight situations on a scale of 0 to 3, with 3 indicating a situation in which chances of dozing off

Table 5.1
Stanford Sleepiness Scale

Wide awake, active, and alert
Awake and able to concentrate but not functioning at peak
Relaxed, awake, and responsive but not fully alert
Feeling a little foggy
Difficulty staying awake
Sleepy, prefer to lie down
Cannot stay awake, sleep onset is imminent

Source: Adapted from E Hoddes, V Zarcone, H Smythe, et al. Quantification of sleepiness: a new approach. Psychophysiology 1973;10:431–436.

are highest. The maximum score is 24 and a score of 10 suggests the presence of excessive sleepiness (Table 5.2). This scale has been weakly correlated with Multiple Sleep Latency Test (MSLT) scores.

The two most important laboratory tests to assess excessive sleepiness are overnight polysomnogram (PSG) and MSLT. The MSLT is an important test for objectively documenting excessive daytime sleepiness and has been standardized.

Technique of the Multiple Sleep Latency Test Procedure

There are several general and specific procedures that are standardized for conducting the MSLT. The guidelines require recording of elec-

Table 5.2
Epworth Sleepiness Scale

Eight Situations	*Scores**
1. Sitting and reading	—
2. Watching television	—
3. Sitting in a public place (e.g., a theater or a meeting)	—
4. Sitting in car as a passenger for an hour without a break	—
5. Lying down to rest in the afternoon	—
6. Sitting and talking to someone	—
7. Sitting quietly after a lunch without alcohol	—
8. In a car, while stopped for a few minutes in traffic	—

*Scale to determine total scores: 0 = would never doze; 1 = slight chance of dozing; 2 = moderate chance of dozing; 3 = high chance of dozing.
Source: Adapted from MW Johns. A new method for measuring daytime sleepiness: the Epworth Sleepiness Scale. Sleep 1991;14:540–545.

troencephalogram (EEG), submental electromyogram (EMG), and electro-oculogram (EOG). In addition to the suggested montage of C3-A2 or C4-A1, it is helpful to add occipital electrodes (O1 and O2, referenced to the ears) to document the alpha activity in relaxed wakefulness and its attenuation or disappearance at the onset of sleep.

General procedures include keeping a sleep diary 1–2 weeks before the test. The sleep diary records information about bedtime, time of rising, napping, and any drug use. Central nervous system (CNS)–active drugs should be discontinued before the test. The test is scheduled approximately 1–3 hours after overnight PSG study. The patient is given breakfast before the study and lunch after the second nap study. The test consists of four to five nap opportunities at 2-hour intervals. Between tests, subjects should be monitored to make certain that they do not fall asleep. Other preparations include smoking cessation 30 minutes before lights out and the completion of electrode connections and calibrations 5 minutes before lights out. The patient is then instructed to relax and fall asleep. The test should be conducted in a quiet, dark room.

The MSLT measures average sleep onset latency and the presence of sleep onset rapid eye movement (SOREM), which is timed from sleep onset to the first rapid eye movement (REM) sleep. For clinical purposes, the nap is concluded 20 minutes after lights out if no sleep occurs and 15 minutes after the first 30-second epoch of any stage of sleep. In case equivocal scoring occurs, it is better to continue the test than to end it prematurely. Mean sleep latency is calculated from the sum of the average latency to sleep onset for each of the naps. A mean sleep latency of less than 5 minutes is consistent with pathologic sleepiness. A mean sleep latency of 10–15 minutes is normal. A mean sleep latency of 5–10 minutes is consistent with mild sleepiness. The occurrence of REM sleep within 15 minutes of sleep onset is defined as SOREM.

Reliability, Validity, and Limitation of the Multiple Sleep Latency Test

The sensitivity and specificity of the MSLT in detecting sleepiness have not been definitely determined. The test–retest reliability of the MSLT has been documented in both normal subjects and patients with narcolepsy. The MSLT has been validated in several studies used to detect pathologic sleepiness, including studies of sleep-deprived normal subjects and studies of sleepiness caused by circadian, hypnotic, and alcohol effects. However, poor correlation exists between the MSLT and Epworth Sleepiness Scale. Interpretation of the MSLT result is also affected by the patient's psychological and behavioral state. The MSLT "unmasks" physiologic sleepiness modulated by circadian rhythm, linked to time of day and homeostatically linked to length of time since morning awakening. Thus, it measures subjects' tendencies to sleep rather than their likelihood of falling asleep. If the patient is psychologically or behaviorally stimulated, the MSLT may not show sleepiness, even in a patient complaining of EDS.

Indications for the Multiple Sleep Latency Test

Narcolepsy is the single most important indication for performing the MSLT. A mean sleep latency of less than 5 minutes, in combination with SOREM in two or more of the four to five recordings during the MSLT, suggests narcolepsy, although abnormalities of the REM sleep regulatory mechanism and circadian rhythm sleep disorders also may lead to such findings. These findings may not be present in a small percentage of narcoleptic patients in the initial MSLT, but on repeating the MSLT, the percentage of positive findings increases considerably.

The MSLT is indicated to assess the degree of severity of daytime sleepiness in patients with obstructive sleep apnea syndrome. Patients sometimes tend to underestimate the presence of sleepiness, and often, denial of daytime symptoms is reported. An MSLT is indicated in patients suspected of having idiopathic hypersomnia, periodic limb movement disorder with EDS, or when the cause of EDS is unknown. In patients with insomnia, MSLT after overnight PSG is indicated when the presence of moderate to severe EDS is suspected.

The usefulness of MSLT in assessing circadian rhythm sleep disorder has not been adequately validated. MSLT is indicated for assessing responses to treatment. The MSLT measures improvement after treatment of narcolepsy by stimulants and of obstructive sleep apnea syndrome by continuous positive airway pressure (CPAP). However, the Maintenance of Wakefulness Test (MWT) may be better for assessing treatment effect in patients with narcolepsy or idiopathic hypersomnia. Adequate outcome studies used to determine MSLT results after treatment of various disorders (causing EDS) need to be performed.

MAINTENANCE OF WAKEFULNESS TEST

The MWT is a variant of the MSLT that measures a patient's ability to stay awake. This test is generally performed at 2-hour intervals in a quiet, dark room. The patient adopts a semireclining position in a chair and is instructed to resist sleep. Four or five such tests are performed; each one lasts either 20 or 40 minutes.

The MWT is useful for differentiating groups with normal daytime alertness from those with EDS. This test has also proved to be sensitive in the assessment of CPAP efficacy in obstructive sleep apnea syndrome and in assessing the effects of stimulant medication treatment in narcolepsy. It is, however, less useful than the MSLT as a diagnostic test for narcolepsy. The MSLT and MWT assess separate functions. The MSLT unmasks physiologic sleepiness determined by circadian and homeostatic factors, whereas the MWT is influenced by physiologic sleepiness and is a reflection of an individual's capability to resist sleep. Each test, therefore, has a unique set of clinical applications. Further studies are needed to test the validity, reliability, and usefulness of MWT.

6

Sleep Scoring Technique

Rechtschaffen and Kales' technique for sleep staging is standard for scoring adult sleep. This is a manual rather than an automated computerized sleep scoring technique. Sleep stage scoring is based on three physiologic criteria: electroencephalography (EEG), electro-oculography (EOG), and electromyography (EMG). For recording techniques used to score these and other physiologic characteristics during an all night polysomnographic (PSG) study, see Chapter 4. For Rechtschaffen and Kales' scoring, an EEG recorded at C3/A2 or C4/A1 should be used, particularly for the purpose of amplitude criteria. An epoch-by-epoch scoring is recommended. The most commonly used is a 30-second epoch. Table 6.1 summarizes sleep-wake scoring criteria in adults.

SCORING CRITERIA FOR WAKEFULNESS

Wakefulness is scored when the EEG shows dominant activity (more than 50% of the epoch) consisting of alpha waves, predominantly in the parieto-occipital region intermixed with low-amplitude fast activity in the beta range. In some people, the dominant activity is low-amplitude fast activities in the beta range. The EMG shows high activity. Frequent waking eye movements intermixed with body movements may occur.

SCORING CRITERIA FOR NONRAPID EYE MOVEMENT STAGE I SLEEP

The transition from wakefulness to stage I is characterized by a reduction of alpha waves or low-amplitude fast activities to less than 50% of the epoch. The EEG is now dominated by low-amplitude fast inter-

Table 6.1
Summary of sleep–wake scoring criteria in adults

Physiologic Characteristics	Awake	Stage I NREM	Stage II NREM	Stage III NREM	Stage IV NREM	REM
Electroencephalogram	Parieto-occipital alpha waves (8–13 Hz) more than 50% of the epoch mixed with fronto-central beta rhythms (>13 Hz)	Alpha waves decrease to less than 50% of the epoch; theta (4–7 Hz) and beta rhythms occur; may have vertex waves	Sleep spindles (approximately 14 Hz) and K complexes lasting at least 0.5 secs; delta waves of 2 Hz or less measuring 75 µV or more occupying <20% of the epoch	Delta waves of 2 Hz or less measuring 75 µV or more occupying 20–50% of the epoch	Delta waves of 2 Hz or less measuring 75 µV or more occupying >50% of the epoch	Theta waves; saw tooth waves; beta rhythms
Electro-oculogram	Waking eye movements	Slow rolling eye movements	Quiescent	Quiescent	Quiescent	REMs
Electromyogram (muscle tone)	Elevated	Elevated but less than in awake stage	Mildly decreased	Mildly decreased	Mildly to moderately decreased	Markedly decreased to absent

NREM = nonrapid eye movement; REM = rapid eye movement.

mixed with theta activities (>3 to <8 Hz). Vertex sharp waves are seen toward the end of stage I. Scoring stage I requires an absolute absence of clearly defined K complexes and sleep spindles lasting for at least 0.5 second. During stage I, slow rolling eye movements may occur, and EMG muscle tone decreases slightly from waking activity.

SCORING CRITERIA FOR NONRAPID EYE MOVEMENT STAGE II SLEEP

The characteristic feature of stage II sleep is the presence of sleep spindles (12–18, most commonly 14 Hz) or a K complex that lasts at least 0.5 second. K complexes are characterized by a well-delineated negative sharp wave followed by a positive component with or without accompanying spindles. The K complex is maximal around the vertex region. K complexes and sleep spindles are transient phenomena and long periods may occur between these events. If the interval between spindles or K complexes is less than 3 minutes, it is scored as stage II. If the interval is 3 minutes or longer, however, its score is stage I. If movement arousal or increases in muscle tone occur during the interval, the portion of the recording that occurs before the movement arousal or increased muscle tone should be scored as stage II. The portion that occurs afterward should be scored as stage I until the next sleep spindles or K complexes are seen. During stage II, the EEG shows delta waves of 2 Hz or slower with amplitudes greater than 75 µV occupying less than 20% of the epoch.

SCORING CRITERIA FOR NONRAPID EYE MOVEMENT STAGE III SLEEP

Nonrapid eye movement (NREM) stage III sleep is defined by an EEG showing delta waves of 2 Hz or slower with amplitudes greater than 75 µV occupying 20–50% of the epoch.

SCORING CRITERIA FOR NONRAPID EYE MOVEMENT STAGE IV SLEEP

Stage IV sleep is scored when the EEG shows delta waves occupying more than 50% of the epoch. Sleep spindles may or may not be present in stage IV. Stage III and stage IV are often combined and called *slow wave sleep*.

SCORING CRITERIA FOR RAPID EYE MOVEMENT SLEEP

During rapid eye movement (REM) sleep, distinctive patterns are seen in the EEG, EMG, and EOG. The EEG shows low-amplitude, mixed-frequency waves resembling those seen in stage I, except that vertex sharp waves are not prominent in REM sleep. Distinctive "saw tooth" waves in vertex and frontal regions may be seen, often heralding the onset of REM sleep. The EOG shows REMs; the EMG shows markedly decreased or absent muscle tone. REM sleep should not be scored in the presence of a relatively elevated tonic EMG. There may be certain problems with scoring at the beginning and end of REM periods because EEG, EOG, and EMG do not necessarily change simultaneously. Occasionally, particularly during the first REM period, sleep spindles are interspersed with REMs. According to scoring rules, any section of record continuous with stage REM in which the EEG shows relatively low-amplitude mixed frequency is scored as REM regardless of whether REMs are present, provided the EMG shows hypotonia or atonia and no intervening arousals occur. An interval of low-amplitude, mixed-frequency EEG between two sleep spindles or K complexes is considered stage II regardless of EMG level if no REMs or arousals occur during the interval and if the interval is less than 3 minutes long.

SCORING OF MOVEMENT TIME, BODY MOVEMENTS, AND MOVEMENT AROUSAL

Movement time (MT) is scored when the EEG and EOG tracings are obscured by muscle action potentials or amplifier-blocking artifacts associated with movements in more than half the epoch. MT should be differentiated from discrete body movements of short durations. Arousals should be differentiated from MT and body movements; the American Sleep Disorders Association (ASDA) has developed guidelines for scoring arousals as described under Scoring of Arousals.

SCORING OF RESPIRATORY EVENTS

Various types of sleep-disordered breathing events (apnea, hypopnea, Cheyne-Stokes respiration) are scored according to the definition provided in Chapter 10. An apnea must be at least 10 seconds in duration for it to be scored. During central apnea, absences of airflow and respiratory effort occur. During obstructive apnea, airflow ceases but respiratory effort continues. During mixed apnea, an initial period of central apnea occurs, followed by obstructive apnea.

SCORING OF PERIODIC LIMB MOVEMENTS IN SLEEP

Periodic limb movements in sleep (PLMS) are counted from the right and left tibialis anterior EMG recordings. PLMS scoring criteria are as follows:

- Must occur as part of four consecutive movements
- Duration of each EMG burst should be 0.5–5.0 seconds
- Interval between bursts should be 4–90 seconds (average interval is 20–40 seconds)
- Amplitude criteria, although somewhat variable, should be at least 25% of the EMG bursts recorded during the pre-sleep calibration recording

Because many, but not all, leg movements may be associated with arousals, the PLMS number should be expressed with and without arousal. The PLMS index is comprised of the number of PLMS that occur per hour of sleep. To be of pathologic significance, the PLMS index should be 5 or more. Respiratory-related leg movements should not be counted as PLMS. PLMS are generally seen during NREM sleep; they are rarely observed during REM sleep.

SCORING OF AROUSALS

Arousals are transient phenomena and result in fragmented sleep rather than in behavioral awakening. The ASDA Task Force has developed preliminary scoring rules for arousal. According to their rules, an EEG arousal is an abrupt shift in EEG frequency that may include alpha, theta, or beta activities but no spindles or delta waves. The subject must be asleep for at least 10 continuous seconds before an EEG arousal can be scored. To score a second arousal, a minimum of 10 continuous seconds of intervening sleep is needed. The EEG frequency shift must be 3–14 seconds in duration. In REM sleep, arousals are scored only when accompanied by concurrent increases in submental EMG amplitude. Arousals in NREM sleep, however, may occur without increases in submental EMG amplitudes. Arousals cannot be scored based on changes in submental EMG amplitude alone. K complexes, delta waves, and artifacts are not counted as arousals unless they are accompanied by frequency shifts. Arousals can also be expressed as an index (number per hour of sleep). Arousal indexes up to 10 can be considered normal.

A representative sample of a polysomnographic report from our laboratory is reproduced in Figure 6.1.

SCORING CRITERIA FOR STATES OF SLEEP AND WAKEFULNESS IN NEWBORN INFANTS

Rechtschaffen and Kales' scoring technique applies to adults, not newborns. Newborn sleep scoring criteria have been outlined by Anders et al. Sleep scoring in children older than 2 years follows Rechtschaffen and Kales' technique. No standardized scoring technique for children between ages newborn and 2 years exists.

In newborns, behavioral and physiologic characteristics are taken into consideration for sleep scoring. As in adults, an epoch-by-epoch approach to coding behavioral and polygraphic patterns is recommended.

Coding of Electroencephalogram

Four patterns of EEG activity that occur during sleep have been described in full-term newborns.

- Low-voltage irregular pattern consists of voltage ranging from 14 to 35 µV; is generally between 20 and 30 µV. The record is dominated by 5–8 Hz activity, but a significant amount of slower activity (1–5 Hz) exists. This pattern is seen in active REM sleep.
- Tracé alternant pattern consists of bursts of high-voltage slow waves (0.5–3 Hz) with occasional rapid low-voltage waves and sharp waves of 2–4 Hz that last for 3–8 seconds and are separated by 4–8 seconds of relative quiescence containing attenuated mixed frequency activities. This pattern is seen specifically in quiet sleep.
- High-voltage slow pattern consists of continuous, moderately rhythmic, medium- to high-voltage recordings with amplitudes of 50–150 µV and frequencies of 0.5–4.0 Hz. This pattern is seen in both quiet and active REM sleep.
- Mixed pattern consists of high- and low-voltage polyrhythmic components. This pattern is also seen in quiet and active REM sleep.

Coding of Respiration

Respiration is coded as a regular or irregular pattern. A regular pattern is coded if the respiratory rate varies less than 20 cycles per minute; an irregular pattern is coded if the rate varies more than 20 cycles per minute.

I. Patient identification
   A. Name
   B. Age and sex
   C. Date of study

II. Introduction
   A. History: The patient, a 60-year-old woman, gives a history of leg discomfort with motor restlessness that has existed since she was 14 years old, which worsens in the evening or when she is lying down. She describes this discomfort as a creepy and tingling sensation between her knees and ankles. She gets relief on rubbing or moving her legs and on walking around the bed. Her clinical history fulfills all of the criteria for diagnosis of RLS. The patient has experienced depression since she was a teenager; she also experiences sleep disturbance in the form of repeated arousals. She tosses and turns in bed, moving her legs throughout the night.
   B. Indication of study: To confirm clinical suspicion of RLS–PLMS disorder.
   C. Past history: Significant past history includes depression and an eating disorder during teenage and young adult years, and hypothyroidism since 1986.
   D. Medications: Patient is on fluoxetine (Prozac), buspirone (BuSpar), and levothyroxine (Synthroid).
   E. Is patient on continuous positive airway pressure or supplemental O_2? No.
   F. Prior surgery: None.

III. Technical description
   A. Total time in bed: 416 mins
   B. Total sleep time: 373.5 mins
   C. PSG recording included
      1. Ten channels of EEG
      2. Two channels of EOG
      3. EMG of chin, right and left tibialis anterior muscles
      4. Airflow by oronasal thermistor
      5. Respiratory effort by thoracoabdominal respiratory bands
      6. O_2 saturation by finger oximetry
      7. Snoring by a microphone
      8. ECG
      9. Body position using a position sensor
     10. Video monitoring
IV. Description of PSG characteristics

Figure 6.1

A representative sample of an overnight polysomnographic (PSG) report. (EEG = electroencephalogram; ECG = electrocardiogram; EMG = electromyogram; EOG = electro-oculogram; NREM = nonrapid eye movement; PLMS = periodic limb movements in sleep; PSG = polysomnograph; REM = rapid eye movement; RLS = restless legs syndrome.)

A. Sleep statistics and architecture
1. Sleep onset latency: 10 mins, which is normal.
2. Sleep efficiency: 89.8%, which is low normal.
3. Sleep stage percentages: stage I NREM sleep, 7.2%; stage II NREM sleep, 61.3%; stage III NREM sleep, 4%; stage IV NREM sleep, 3.3%; and REM sleep, 24.2%. Thus, the patient shows slightly increased stage II NREM sleep and markedly decreased slow wave sleep.
4. REM sleep latency: 153 minutes, which is prolonged.
5. Number of REM cycles: four. The first cycle has the shortest and the last cycle has the longest duration.
B. Respiratory events: The patient has three central apneas during NREM sleep, giving rise to an apnea-hypopnea index of 0.5, which is well within the normal range.
C. Snoring: No significant snoring is noted.
D. ECG: No cardiac arrhythmias are noted.
E. PLMS: The patient has a total of 426 PLMS, giving rise to a PLMS index of 68.4, which is markedly increased. The PLMS index without arousal is 58, which is also markedly increased; the PLMS index with arousal is 10.4, which is only slightly increased.
F. O_2 saturation: O_2 saturation stays approximately 96–98% and, thus, the patient does not show any O_2 desaturation.
G. EEG characteristics: The sleep EEG characteristics have been described under "Sleep statistics and architecture." No epileptiform discharges are seen. The patient has a total of 105 arousals, giving rise to an arousal index of 16.9, which is slightly increased. All the arousals are associated with PLMS.
H. Behavioral data: Nothing significant.

V. Summary and impression

The overnight PSG study is abnormal because of a markedly increased PLMS index, most of which is not associated with arousal. No evidence of sleep apnea-hypopnea syndrome exists. In conjunction with the clinical description of symptoms, these PSG findings are consistent with a diagnosis of RLS–PLMS disorder.

Figure 6.1 Continued.

Coding of Eye Movements

Eye movements are coded positive if a single REM or bursts of REM are present within an epoch; they are coded negative if no REMs are present.

Coding of Electromyogram

EMG is coded high if more than half of the epoch is occupied by tonic muscle activity; it is coded low if more than half of the epoch shows muscle suppression.

Table 6.2
Newborn and infant awake scoring criteria

Behavioral pattern: eyes open; vocalization; body movements
Electroencephalogram: mixed slow-wave pattern with predominantly theta
   (4–7 Hz) waves with some delta (<4 Hz) and beta (>13 Hz) waves
Electro-oculogram: waking eye movements
Electromyogram: sustained tonic electromyogram with phasic bursts
Respiration: variable rate

Table 6.3
Newborn and infant active rapid eye movement sleep scoring criteria

Behavioral pattern: eyes closed but visible movements; smiles, facial grimaces,
   limb and gross body movements; vocalization
Electroencephalogram: low-voltage irregular or mixed polyrhythmic waves
Electro-oculogram: positive with rapid eye movements
Electromyogram: low or absent muscle tone
Respiration: irregular with variation greater than 20 breaths/min

Table 6.4
Newborn and infant quiet sleep scoring criteria

Behavioral pattern: eyes closed; behavioral quiescence; no body movements
   except for occasional startles and mouth movements
Electroencephalogram: high-voltage slow waves, mixed pattern or tracé alter-
   nant (bursts of slow waves interspersed with periods of relative quiescence)
Electro-oculogram: negative (quiescent)
Electromyogram: high (elevated tone)
Respiration: regular (variation less than 20 breaths/min)

Tables 6.2, 6.3, and 6.4 list criteria for scoring awake, active REM sleep and quiet sleep in newborns. Certain epochs do not meet all active REM sleep or quiet sleep criteria. These epochs should be scored as *indeterminate sleep*. In normal newborns, such indeterminate or transitional epochs occur most often at sleep onset, during times of state changing, and infant arousing.

7

Classification and Approach to a Patient with Sleep Disorders

The original diagnostic classification of sleep and arousal disorders by the Association of Sleep Disorders Centers divided sleep–wake disorders into four classes: (1) disorders of initiating and maintaining sleep; (2) disorders of excessive somnolence; (3) disorders of sleep–wake schedule; and (4) dysfunctions associated with sleep, sleep stages, or partial arousals. This classification has been supplanted by the 1990 International Classification of Sleep Disorders (ICSD), which was revised slightly in 1997. The ICSD system, used by sleep specialists, lists 84 sleep disorders in four broad categories: (1) dyssomnias, (2) parasomnias, (3) sleep disorders associated with medical or psychiatric disorders, and (4) proposed sleep disorders (Table 7.1).

Dyssomnias are disorders that produce difficulty initiating or maintaining sleep or excessive sleepiness. Dyssomnias are subdivided to include intrinsic, extrinsic, and circadian rhythm sleep disorders. Intrinsic disorders result from bodily causes, whereas extrinsic disorders are primarily caused by environmental factors. Circadian rhythm disorders result from disruption of sleep–wake schedule changes.

Parasomnias are characterized by abnormal movements and behavior during sleep that do not necessarily disrupt sleep architecture. Parasomnias consist of arousal and sleep–wake transition disorders, rapid eye movement (REM)–related parasomnias, and other disorders.

Medical or psychiatric disorders include those attributable to other conditions; they are secondary to psychiatric, neurologic, and other medical disorders.

Proposed sleep disorders include those whose existence is unable to be substantiated with certainty because adequate or sufficient information is unavailable.

The ICSD includes descriptive details, specific diagnostic, severity, and duration criteria, as well as an axial system for standardizing clinical presentations of relevant information about patient disorders.

Table 7.1
International Classification of Sleep Disorders

Dyssomnias	Parasomnias	Sleep Disorders Associated with Medical/Psychiatric Disorders	Proposed Sleep Disorders
Intrinsic sleep disorders	Arousal disorders	Mental disorders	Short sleeper
Psychophysiologic insomnia	Confusional insomnia	Psychoses	Long sleeper
Sleep state misperception	Sleepwalking	Mood disorders	Subwakefulness syndrome
Idiopathic insomnia	Sleep terrors	Anxiety disorders	Fragmentary myoclonus
Narcolepsy	Sleep–wake transition disorders	Panic disorders	Sleep hyperhidrosis
Recurrent hypersomnia	Rhythmic movement disorder	Alcoholism	Menstrual-associated sleep disorder
Idiopathic hypersomnia	Sleep starts	Neurologic disorders	Pregnancy-associated sleep disorder
Obstructive sleep apnea syndrome	Sleep talking	Cerebral degenerative disorders	Terrifying hypnagogic hallucinations
Central sleep apnea syndrome	Nocturnal leg cramps	Dementia	Sleep-related neurogenic tachypnea
Central alveolar hypoventilation syndrome	Parasomnias usually associated with rapid eye movement (REM) sleep	Parkinsonism	Sleep-related laryngospasm
Periodic limb movements in sleep disorder	Nightmares	Fatal familial insomnia	Sleep choking syndrome
Restless legs syndrome	Sleep paralysis	Sleep-related epilepsy	
Intrinsic sleep disorders not otherwise specified	Impaired sleep-related penile erections	Electrical status epilepticus of sleep	
Extrinsic sleep disorders	Sleep-related painful erections	Sleep-related headaches	
Inadequate sleep hygiene	REM sleep–related sinus arrest	Other medical disorders	
Environmental sleep disorder		Sleeping sickness	
Altitude insomnia		Nocturnal cardiac ischemia	
Adjustment sleep disorder		Chronic obstructive pulmonary disease	
Insufficient sleep disorder			

Limit-setting sleep disorder
Sleep-onset association disorder
Food allergy insomnia
Nocturnal eating (drinking) syndrome
Hypnotic-dependent sleep disorder
Stimulant-dependent sleep disorder
Alcohol-dependent sleep disorder
Toxin-induced sleep disorder
Extrinsic sleep disorders not otherwise specified
Circadian rhythm sleep disorders
Time-zone (jet lag) syndrome
Shift-work sleep disorder
Irregular sleep-wake pattern disorder
Delayed-sleep-phase syndrome
Non–24-hr sleep–wake disorder
Advanced sleep phase syndrome
Circadian rhythm sleep disorders not otherwise specified

REM sleep behavior disorder
Other parasomnias
Sleep bruxism
Sleep enuresis
Sleep-related abnormal swallowing syndrome
Nocturnal paroxysmal dystonia
Sudden unexplained nocturnal death syndrome
Primary snoring
Infant sleep apnea
Congenital central hypoventilation syndrome
Sudden infant death syndrome
Benign neonatal sleep myoclonus
Other parasomnias not otherwise specified

Sleep-related asthma
Sleep-related gastroesophageal reflux
Peptic ulcer disease
Fibromyalgia

Axis A contains the primary sleep diagnosis of the ICSD. Axis B lists tests and procedures performed in the practice of sleep medicine (e.g., all-night polysomnography [PSG] and Multiple Sleep Latency Test [MSLT]). Axis C consists of medical and psychiatric disorders that are not primarily sleep disorders. The ICSD also contains coding information for clinical and research purposes.

Several other classification systems also exist: the *International Classification of Diseases, Ninth Revision, Clinical Modification* (*ICD-9-CM*) and the *ICD, Tenth Revision* (*ICD-10*). The *ICD-10-Alphanumeric* is an expansion of the *ICD-10* that contains alphanumeric codes for every neurologic disease, including specific sleep disorders. No study has been conducted to assess the validity and reliability of any of these sleep disorder classification systems.

APPROACH TO PATIENTS WITH SLEEP COMPLAINTS

Treating patients with sleep complaints requires a clear understanding of sleep disorders as they are listed in the ICSD. Some common sleep complaints are trouble falling and staying asleep (insomnia), falling asleep during the day (daytime hypersomnolence), and the inability to sleep at the right time (circadian rhythm sleep disorders) (Table 7.2). Other common complaints include thrashing or moving about in bed with repeated leg jerking (i.e., parasomnias and other abnormal movements, including nocturnal seizures and restless legs syndrome [RLS]). Cardinal manifestations in a patient complaining of insomnia (Table 7.3) include some or all of the following: difficulty falling asleep, frequent awakenings (including early morning awakening), insufficient or total lack of sleep, daytime fatigue, and tiredness or sleepiness, lack of concentration, irritability, anxiety, depression, forgetfulness, and preoccupation with psychosomatic symptoms such as aches and pains.

Table 7.2
Common sleep complaints

Cannot sleep (trouble falling asleep and staying asleep)
Cannot stay awake (falling asleep during the day)
Cannot sleep at the right time
Thrash and move about in bed and experience repeated leg jerking

---

Table 7.3
Cardinal manifestations of insomnia

Difficulty falling asleep
Frequent awakenings
Early morning awakening
Insufficient sleep
Daytime fatigue or sleepiness
Lack of concentration or irritability
Anxiety, sometimes depression
Forgetfulness
Psychosomatic symptoms

Cardinal manifestations of hypersomnia (Table 7.4) include excessive daytime somnolence (EDS) and falling asleep in inappropriate places or under inappropriate circumstances (see Chapter 5). The patient experiences no relief of symptoms after additional sleep at night or after taking a nap; he or she experiences daytime fatigue, inability to concentrate, and impairment of motor skills and cognition. Additional symptoms depend on the nature of the underlying sleep disorder (e.g., snoring and apneas during sleep in patients with obstructive sleep apnea syndrome [OSAS], attacks of cataplexy, hypnagogic hallucination or sleep paralysis, and automatic behavior and disturbed night sleep in patients with narcolepsy).

Insomnia and EDS are themselves symptoms; every attempt should be made to find causes for these complaints. Insomnia may be secondary to a variety of causes (see Chapter 11). EDS may result from physiologic and pathologic causes (Table 7.5). Sleep deprivation and sleepiness secondary to lifestyle or irregular sleep and waking habits

Table 7.4
Cardinal manifestations of hypersomnia

Excessive daytime somnolence
Falling asleep in inappropriate places and circumstances
Lack of relief of symptoms after additional sleep
Daytime fatigue
Inability to concentrate
Impairment of motor skills and cognition
Symptoms specific to etiology (e.g., sleep apnea, narcolepsy)

Table 7.5
Causes of excessive daytime somnolence

Physiologic causes
    Sleep deprivation and sleepiness related to lifestyle and irregular
        sleep–wake schedule
Pathologic causes
    Primary sleep disorders
        Obstructive sleep apnea syndrome
        Central sleep apnea syndrome
        Narcolepsy
        Idiopathic hypersomnolence
        Circadian rhythm sleep disorders
            Jet lag
            Delayed sleep phase syndrome
            Irregular sleep–wake pattern
            Shift work sleep disorder
            Non–24-hr sleep–wake disorders
        Periodic limb movements in sleep disorder
        Restless legs syndrome
        Insufficient sleep syndrome
        Inadequate sleep hygiene
        Recurrent or periodic hypersomnia
            Kleine-Levin syndrome
            Idiopathic recurrent stupor
            Catamenial hypersomnia
            Seasonal affective depression
            Occasionally secondary to insomnia
   General medical disorders
        Hepatic failure
        Renal failure
        Respiratory failure
        Electrolyte disturbances
        Cardiac failure
        Severe anemia
        Endocrine causes
            Hypothyroidism
            Acromegaly
            Diabetes mellitus
            Hypoglycemia
            Hyperglycemia
Psychiatric or psychological causes
    Depression
    Psychogenic unresponsiveness or sleepiness
Neurologic causes
    Brain tumors or vascular lesions affecting thalamus, hypothalamus, or
        brain stem
    Post-traumatic hypersomnolence
    Multiple sclerosis

Encephalitis lethargica and other encephalitides and encephalopathies, including Wernicke's encephalopathy
Cerebral trypanosomiasis ("African sleeping sickness")
Neurodegenerative disorders
   Alzheimer's disease
   Parkinson's disease
   Multiple system atrophy
Myotonic dystrophy and other neuromuscular disorders causing sleepiness secondary to sleep apnea
Medication-related hypersomnia
   Benzodiazepines
   Nonbenzodiazepine hypnotics (e.g., phenobarbital, zolpidem)
   Sedative antidepressants (e.g., tricyclics, trazodone)
   Antipsychotics
   Nonbenzodiazepine anxiolytics (e.g., buspirone)
   Antihistamines
   Narcotic analgesics, including tramadol (Ultram)
   Beta blockers
Toxin- and alcohol-induced hypersomnolence

can be considered physiologic causes of EDS, resulting from disruptions in normal circadian and homeostatic physiology. Groups of people who often are excessively sleepy because of lifestyle or inadequate sleep include young adults and elderly individuals, people who work irregular shifts, health care professionals, firefighters, police officers, train engineers, pilots, flight attendants, commercial truck drivers, and anyone with a competitive drive to move ahead in life who sacrifices hours of sleep and accumulates sleep debt. High school and college students are particularly at risk for sleep deprivation and sleepiness. Biological and psychosocial factors contribute to excessive sleepiness, but the role biological factors play is not well studied. For example, teenagers need extra hours of sleep, and the circadian timing system may change with sleep phase delays in teenagers. Pathologic causes of sleepiness as listed in Table 7.5 are described in Chapters 10 and 12–17.

Clinical Evaluation

The physician must first evaluate the patient based on history and physical examination before undertaking laboratory tests, which must be subservient to the clinical diagnosis (Table 7.6). The first step in assessing a sleep–wakefulness disturbance is careful evaluation of sleep

Table 7.6
Clinical evaluation of a patient with sleep complaints

History
    Sleep history
    Sleep questionnaire
    Sleep log or diary
    Drug and alcohol history
    Psychiatric history
    General medical history
    Neurologic history
    History of previous illnesses
    Family history
Physical examination

---

complaints. Patient history should include information about sleep habits; drug use; alcohol consumption; psychiatric, medical, and neurologic illnesses; history of previous illness; and family history.

Sleep histories must encompass entire 24-hour spans, not just symptoms occurring at sleep onset or during sleep at night. Clinicians should pay attention to symptoms that occur in the early evening or at sleep onset (e.g., paresthesia and uncomfortable limb movements of RLS), during sleep at night (e.g., repeated awakenings, snoring, and cessation of breathing in OSAS), on awakening in the morning (e.g., feeling exhausted and sleepy as in OSAS), or in late morning and afternoon (e.g., daytime fatigue and excessive somnolence as in OSAS, an irresistible desire to a brief sleep as in narcolepsy). Early morning awakening may be noted in insomnia due to depression. Abnormal motor activities may be associated with REM sleep behavior disorder, other parasomnias, and seizure disorders.

Understanding patient problems requires consideration of psychological, social, medical, and biological factors and how they interact. The physician should inquire about the patient's functional status and mood during the day and any medication the patient is taking that may have effects on sleep complaint and sleep hygiene. An interview with the patient's bed partner and caregiver (or, in the case of a child, a parent), is important for diagnosing abnormal movements (PLMS or other body movements), abnormal behavior (parasomnias, nocturnal seizures), and breathing disorders during sleep. The bed partner may also be able to answer questions about the patient's sleeping habits, history of drug use, psychosocial problems (e.g., stress at home, work, or school), and changes in his or her sleep habits. Patients may fill out a sleep questionnaire containing a list of pertinent questions relating to sleep complaints to save time (e.g., sleep hygiene, sleep patterns, medical, psychiatric, and neurologic disorders, drug and alcohol use).

A sleep log or diary kept over a 2-week period is also a valuable indicator of sleep hygiene. Such a log should document bedtime, arising time, and daytime nap information; amount of time needed to go to sleep; number of nighttime awakenings; total sleep time; and feelings on arousal (e.g., whether the patient is refreshed or drowsy). Questions should also be asked regarding the patient's mood and naps taken during the daytime. In women, the relation of insomnia and sleepiness to their menstrual cycles should also be ascertained.

Family history is important in certain sleep disorders. Approximately one-third of patients with narcolepsy and RLS has a family history of sleep disorders. OSAS, with or without obesity, has also been described as affecting other family members. Prevalence of sleep walking, sleep terrors, and primary enuresis in other family members is high. Many neurologic disorders, including fatal familial insomnia, have family histories.

A careful physical examination is important and may uncover various medical disorders such as respiratory, cardiovascular, endocrine, or neurologic disorders, especially those affecting the brain stem region or neuromuscular system. Physical examination in OSAS may uncover upper airway anatomic abnormalities that require surgical correction if medical and continuous positive airway pressure (CPAP) treatment fail to relieve symptoms. Examination may reveal systemic hypertension, a risk factor for sleep apnea.

Several scales have been developed to assess subjective measurements of sleepiness. These are described in Chapter 5.

Laboratory Assessment

Laboratory tests should include diagnostic work-up for the primary condition causing secondary sleep disturbance and work-up for the sleep disturbance itself (Table 7.7).

The two most important laboratory tests for diagnosis of sleep disturbances are PSG study and MSLT (see Chapters 4 and 5). Other tests (e.g., Maintenance of Wakefulness Test [MWT], actigraphy, video-PSG study, standard electroencephalography [EEG], 24-hour ambulatory EEG recording, and long-term video EEG monitoring) are also important for assessing patients with sleep dysfunctions. These various tests are described in Chapters 4, 5, 10, and 14.

An overnight PSG study is the single most important laboratory test for diagnosing and treating patients with EDS. MSLT is an important

Table 7.7
Laboratory assessment

Diagnostic workup for the primary condition causing secondary sleep
   disturbance
Laboratory tests for the diagnosis of sleep disorder
   Overnight polysomnographic (PSG) study
   Multiple sleep latency test
   Maintenance of wakefulness test
   Actigraphy
   Video-PSG
Standard electroencephalography (EEG)
Video-EEG monitoring
Neuroimaging study in cases of suspected neurologic illness causing sleep
   disorders
Pulmonary function tests in cases of suspected bronchopulmonary diseases
   causing sleep apnea

---

test for objectively documenting excessive sleepiness and sleep onset
rapid eye movements (SOREMs). A mean sleep latency of less than 5
minutes, which is consistent with pathologic sleepiness in conjunction
with SOREMs in two or more of the four to five recordings during
MSLT, strongly suggests narcolepsy. The MWT is a variant of the MSLT
that measures a patient's ability to stay awake. This test is important
for monitoring the effect of treatment in narcolepsy, but it is not as
good as MSLT for measuring daytime sleepiness. Actigraphy is a technique of motion detection that records activities during sleep and waking. It complements sleep log or diary data and is useful in diagnosing
circadian rhythm sleep disorders.

Video-PSG study is important for documenting abnormal movements and behaviors that occur during nighttime sleep in patients with
parasomnias, including REM sleep behavior disorder, nocturnal
seizures, and other unusual movements. Parasomnias are generally
diagnosed on the basis of clinical history, but sometimes video-PSG is
required to document these conditions. Standard EEG as well as 24-
hour ambulatory EEG recordings and long-term video EEG monitoring may be needed for the documentation of seizures in some cases.

Neuroimaging study is essential when a neurologic illness is suspected of causing a sleep disturbance. Pulmonary function tests are
important for excluding intrinsic bronchopulmonary disease, which
may affect sleep-related breathing disorders (see Chapter 14). Other
appropriate laboratory tests should always be performed to exclude any

suspected medical disorders that may be the cause of patients' insomnia or hypersomnia.

SUMMARY AND CONCLUSION

The approach to treating patients with sleep complaints should begin with a careful clinical analysis of patient symptoms. A detailed history consisting of the patient's sleep history as well as family, psychiatric, medical (including neurologic), drug, and alcohol histories should be taken. Physical examination should include neurologic and general medical and other organ system examinations. Keeping a sleep diary or log is often useful. An occasional sleep complaint (insomnia or sleepiness) is common, but if symptoms are persistent or frequent and interfere with daily life, professional advice should be sought. In most cases, a diagnosis can be made on clinical grounds with minimal laboratory investigation, minimizing patient suffering and expense. In this way, the Hippocratic oath is honored by comforting patients and causing no harm. Most of the time, patients with sleep complaints seek the advice of their primary care physicians, who may decide, based on patient history and physical examination, that their patients' sleep complaints are owing to medical, psychiatric, or neurologic conditions. The next step for the primary care physician is either to treat the condition causing the sleep disturbance or refer the patient to an appropriate specialist. For primary sleep disorders, it is advisable to refer patients to sleep specialists, who may then decide to conduct further laboratory tests (e.g., PSG, MSLT, actigraphy, or video-PSG) and provide treatment.

8

Epidemiology of Sleep Disorders

Despite the considerable progress that has been made in understanding and classifying sleep disorders, progress in the field of epidemiology of sleep disorders has been slow. Difficulties involving definitions and diagnostic criteria of various sleep disorders, as well as difficulties in confirming clinical diagnoses through large-scale polysomnographic (PSG) studies in the population, have contributed to this slow progress. Many studies are based on well-designed questionnaires; some are based on PSG and other laboratory tests. This chapter briefly reviews the epidemiologic surveys that exist for the following categories of sleep disorders: insomnia, excessive sleepiness, snoring, sleep-disordered breathing, and parasomnias.

EPIDEMIOLOGY OF INSOMNIA

Insomnia is the most common sleep disorder in the United States. It is experienced at some time by approximately one-third of the U.S. adult population and is a persistent problem in approximately 10%. Surveys have been conducted in North America and western Europe (Table 8.1). One of the earliest surveys was conducted in metropolitan Los Angeles and involved more than 1,000 subjects, age 18 years or older. Insomnia complaints were noted in 32.2% of the subjects. In another large-scale epidemiologic study conducted in the San Francisco Bay Area, 31% of the 6,340 subjects surveyed complained of insomnia. A 1979 study by Mellinger et al. involving 3,161 individuals, 18–79 years of age, found the 12-month prevalence of insomnia to be 35%. In the National Institute of Mental Health Epidemiologic Catchment Area study conducted between 1981 and 1985, the 6-month prevalence of insomnia was 10.2% in a sample of 7,954 respondents, age 18 years or older. Insomnia complaints were associated with a higher risk of developing depression within the next 12 months. In a more recent

Table 8.1
Epidemiology of insomnia

Survey (yr)	Prevalence (%)
Los Angeles survey (1972)	32.2
San Francisco Bay Area survey (1983)	31
Mellinger et al. (1979)	35
National Institute of Mental Health Epidemiologic Catchment Area survey (Ford and Kamerow) (1981–1985)	10.2 (high risk of depression)
Montreal metropolitan area survey (1997)	29
Swedish survey (1984–1985)	21.2 (sleep initiation)
	22.4 (sleep maintenance)
United Kingdom survey (1997)	36.2

survey conducted in the Montreal metropolitan area, the prevalence of insomnia was 29% in a sample of 1,722 people, ages 15–100 years.

In western Europe, important surveys have been conducted in the San Marino area of Italy, Iceland, Norway, Sweden, France, and the United Kingdom. In a 1984–1985 survey, Gislason and Almqvist, using a sample of 3,201 Swedish men, ages 30–69 years, found a prevalence of 6.9% for severe insomnia and 14.3% for moderate sleep-initiating insomnia. Sleep maintenance insomnia was observed in 7.5% in the severe category and 14.9% in the moderate category. In the large United Kingdom survey involving 4,972 subjects, 36.2% had at least one insomnia symptom.

Most of the surveys noted that prevalence of insomnia increases with age and that symptoms are more common in women than in men. Higher prevalences of insomnia occur in persons of lower socio-economic status, divorced, widowed, or separated individuals, and those with recent stress, depression, drug, or alcohol abuse. An increased association with general medical complaints also exists. One difficulty that has been encountered in all of these surveys is the failure to achieve a standardized definition of insomnia.

EPIDEMIOLOGY OF EXCESSIVE SLEEPINESS

The absence of a consistent definition for excessive sleepiness has also been a confounding factor in various surveys, producing wide variations in the prevalence of excessive daytime somnolence (EDS) (Table

Table 8.2
Epidemiology of excessive daytime somnolence (EDS)

Survey (yr)	Prevalence (%)
Four U.S. surveys (1976–1996)	0.3–16.3
Swedish survey (1987)	16.7 (moderate EDS)
Finnish survey (1996)	9
Swedish survey (1996)	32.0 in men; 23.2 in women
United Kingdom study (1997)	15.2 (moderate EDS)

8.2). In four U.S. surveys measuring hypersomnia, wide variation (from 0.3% to 16.3%) exists. No gender differences were found, but rates were highest in youngest age groups. In one survey that included a sample of 3,962 elderly community subjects, the mortality risk associated with EDS was increased in those who napped most of the time or who made two or more errors on a cognitive test. EDS was found more commonly in overweight men. This survey supports earlier studies that found both "long" and "short" sleepers to have higher mortality risks than the rest of the population.

In the western European studies, most EDS surveys have been conducted in Nordic countries (i.e., Iceland, Finland, and Sweden). Gislason and Almqvist reported a moderate EDS prevalence of 16.7% and a major EDS prevalence of 5.7%. Hublin et al. found a 9% prevalence of EDS in Finnish twin cohorts. Depression was noted in one-fourth of those complaining of sleepiness; narcolepsy was found in 0.3%. In an important study among the elderly members of a community of 6,143 subjects, 32.0% of men and 23.2% of women complained of excessive sleepiness during the day. Sleepiness increased with age and was associated with poor sleep, somatic disease, and poor health status. In a United Kingdom study, Ohayon et al. found severe daytime sleepiness occurring in 5.5% of those surveyed, with moderate daytime sleepiness occurring in 15.2%. They also found increased associations between EDS and mood disorders, psychophysiologic insomnia, obstructive sleep apnea syndrome (OSAS), restless legs syndrome, and insufficient sleep syndrome. Narcolepsy was found in 0.04% of those surveyed and idiopathic hypersomnia was found in 0.20%.

Several general conclusions can be made based on these surveys. Unlike insomnia, EDS is not gender-related. EDS can be a primary symptom of idiopathic hypersomnia or narcolepsy, which has a prevalence rate of only 0.026–0.040%. In all of the surveys, EDS is associated with sleep-disordered breathing, psychiatric disorders (particularly

Table 8.3
Epidemiology of snoring

Survey (yr)	Prevalence (%)
San Marino survey (1981)	19 (habitual snorers); 60 in subjects age 60 yrs and older
British survey (1993)	37
Finnish survey (1994)	20.4 (frequent snorers)
Danish survey (1995)	49.9

depression), and physical ailments, as well as several lifestyle factors, such as work conditions, poor sleep hygiene, and psychotropic drug use.

EPIDEMIOLOGY OF SNORING

In all surveys conducted (Table 8.3), snoring prevalence is found to be higher among men than women and to increase with age. In the San Marino survey, Lugaresi et al. found that 19% of 5,713 subjects were habitual snorers; the rate increased to 60% in those age 60 years or older. In a British survey consisting of a random sample of 1,478 people, age 18 years or older, snoring was found in 37% of the sample. Frequent snoring alone was found in 11%. The study confirmed that snoring is most prevalent in men and older subjects. In a Finnish survey of 3,750 men, 40–59 years of age, 8.8% were habitual snorers and 20.4% were frequent snorers. Snoring was associated with increased body mass index (i.e., being overweight or obese), smoking, physical inactivity, hostility, and morning tiredness. Two important studies attempted to identify mortality risks for snorers. A Danish survey of 2,937 men, ages 54–74 years, conducted over a 6-year period reported snoring (always or often) in 49.9%. These authors found no increased mortality rate in snorers than in nonsnorers and found equal risks of ischemic heart disease in snorers and nonsnorers. A Finnish 5-year follow-up study that surveyed 1,190 participants, ages 36–50 years, found a higher incidence of dozing off at the wheel among habitual snorers than among nonsnorers.

EPIDEMIOLOGY OF SLEEP APNEA

In suspected cases of OSAS, PSG recording is necessary to confirm diagnoses. From a practical point of view, however, it is not possible to con-

Table 8.4
Epidemiology of sleep apnea

Survey (yr)	Prevalence (%)
Israel study (1983)	2.7 (AHI ≥10)
Finnish twin study (1987)	1.4 (AHI ≥10)
Swedish survey (1988)	0.9 (AHI ≥10)
	1.5 (AHI ≥5)
Wisconsin cohort study (1993)	4 in men; 2 in women (EDS; AHI ≥5)

AHI = apnea–hypopnea index; EDS = excessive daytime somnolence.

duct PSG studies in large population samples; therefore, a wide variation exists in reported prevalences of OSAS, depending on whether a
study is based on the questionnaire or PSG study (Table 8.4).

A study of 300 working men was conducted in Israel by Lavie; 78 of
the subjects had PSG performed. In 2.7% of the sample, the
apnea–hypopnea index (AHI) was equal to or greater than 10; in 0.7%,
it was equal to or greater than 20. In a later Finnish twin cohort study
of 278 men, ages 41–50 years, PSG recordings were obtained for 25
snorers and 27 nonsnorers. Researchers found AHIs greater than or
equal to 10 in 1.4% of subjects and AHIs greater than or equal to 20
in 0.4%. Gislason et al. surveyed 3,201 Swedish men, 30–60 years of
age, including 61 men with EDS and snoring who had PSG recordings.
Investigators found AHIs greater than or equal to 10 in 0.9% of subjects and greater than or equal to 5 in 1.5%.

The Wisconsin Sleep Cohort Study surveyed 3,513 workers, ages
30–60 years. Its authors performed one-night PSG recording on 625
subjects, including all those subjects who were habitual snorers as well
as 25% who were nonhabitual snorers. In that study, the prevalence
of sleep apnea syndrome defined as EDS associated with AHIs greater
than or equal to 5 was 4% in men and 2% in women.

No satisfactory surveys have been conducted to determine the true
prevalence of OSAS in the general population. Perhaps the most serious flaw in the surveys was that most were cohort studies. A PSG study
in a true random sample of subjects is needed.

EPIDEMIOLOGY OF PARASOMNIAS

Parasomnias are sleep disorders characterized by the intrusion of
abnormal behaviors or movements during sleep or during sleep–wake

transitions. No adequate studies of parasomnias have been conducted in the general population. Arousal disorders (i.e., sleep walking, sleep terror, and confusional arousals) occur primarily during childhood and rarely persist in adulthood. In children, the prevalence of sleep terror ranges from 1.0% to 6.5%. In the general adult population, the prevalence of sleep walking ranges from 0.5% to 3.0%. Infrequent (less than monthly) episodes were reported by 3.2% of men and 2.6% of women.

Only a few surveys are available for sleep–wake transition disorders. Sleep talking is frequent in younger age groups, in which 3.0% report frequent sleep talking and 21.3% report infrequent sleep talking. The prevalence of nocturnal leg cramps is not well known but appears to be frequent among elderly subjects and subjects with severe daytime sleepiness.

The prevalence of rapid eye movement sleep behavior disorder in the general population is not well documented. Nightmares, which are other rapid eye movement sleep parasomnias, have been reported to occur at least once a week in approximately 5% of the adult population.

In one study, the prevalence of sleep paralysis was estimated to be 11.3%.

9

Genetics of Sleep
and Sleep Disorders

Limited studies of the molecular genetics of normal human sleep and sleep disorders are available. Sleep habits depend on genetic and environmental factors. Most twin studies are based on questionnaires; only a few are based on polysomnographic (PSG) recordings. Furthermore, circadian and homeostatic factors were not considered in the majority of early studies seeking to understand the genetic influence of sleep habits on the general population.

Genetic studies of sleep disorders, particularly narcolepsy, took a significant leap in 1983 when Honda et al. showed associations between HLA and narcolepsy in 100% of narcoleptic Japanese subjects.

GENETIC ASPECTS OF NARCOLEPSY

Approximately 1–2% of the first-degree relatives of narcoleptic patients manifest the illness, compared with 0.02–0.18% in the general population, a prevalence 10 to 40 times higher than that existing in the general population. Early studies of positive family history of hypersomnolence (and, less commonly, of cataplexy) in up to 50% of relatives of narcoleptic patients were based on symptoms only rather than PSG studies; therefore, cases of sleep apnea causing excessive daytime somnolence (EDS) may have been misdiagnosed as narcolepsy. Some reports show that 4.7% of first-degree relatives of narcoleptic or cataplectic patients complain of EDS. The prevalence of EDS in the general population may be approximately 13%; hence, it can be concluded that most sleepy relatives of narcoleptic patients do not have narcolepsy.

Twin studies of narcolepsy document a lack of strong genetic influence. The majority of monozygotic twins are discordant for narcolepsy; only 25–31% are concordant, suggesting an influence of environmental factors in the etiology of narcolepsy. Furthermore, the identification of three discordant dizygotic twins in a sample of 11,354 twins in the Finnish study suggests that an interaction between environmental and genetic factors plays a role in the development of narcolepsy.

DR15 subtype of DR2 haplotypes and DQ6 subtype of DQ1 haplotypes are closely associated with narcolepsy in 95–100% of cases in white and Japanese patients. In African-Americans with narcolepsy, DR2 antigen is found in only 65%; however, DQ1 is present in more than 90% of cases. HLA DQB1*0602 has been established as the narcolepsy subtype gene along with allele DQA1*0102, located nearby on chromosome 6 across all ethnic groups. It should be remembered, however, that cases of narcolepsy not carrying HLA-DR2 or DQ1 antigens have been reported. Furthermore, 12–38% of the general population carry the same HLA alleles but narcolepsy is present in only 0.02–0.18% of the population. Therefore, the alleles DQB1*0602 and DQA1*0102 are neither necessary nor sufficient for development of narcolepsy.

Because it is associated with HLA, autoimmunity in narcolepsy has been questioned, but no definite evidence has been uncovered. Also, neither exact environmental factors nor genetic factors of narcolepsy are known.

The mode of inheritance of narcolepsy is thought to be autosomal dominant in humans, recessive in Doberman pinschers (canarc-1) and Labrador retrievers, and multifactorial in poodles. The canine narcoleptic gene has recently been located in association with hypocretin in the lateral hypothalamic neurons.

GENETIC STUDIES OF RESTLESS LEGS SYNDROME

Up to one-third of restless legs syndrome (RLS) cases are transmitted as autosomal-dominant traits. No twin studies exist for RLS. Linkage studies using either microsatellite markers or candidate genes in multiplex families to identify involved genes are ongoing in a few centers, but no definite linkage has been established yet. The search for candidate genes is suggested by therapeutic results. Pharmacologic treatment suggests possible neurotransmitter involvement, particularly of those involving dopaminergic or peptidergic metabolism in RLS pathogenesis. It is important to find out whether candidate genes involve the enzymes and receptors of these two neurotransmitters.

Some observations of higher prevalence of RLS in patients with Charcot-Marie-Tooth neuronal type (CMT2) and in autosomal-dominant spinocerebellar ataxia (SCA3 type) suggest genetic and phenotypic heterogeneity in RLS.

No population-based risk estimates exist for first- and second-degree relatives of RLS patients, except for a study conducted by Johns Hopkins University and the University of Texas Southwestern Medical Center. In this study, the authors compared rates of RLS in 96 patients to those in relatives of 15 control subjects. Samples included 592 first-degree relatives and 1,518 second-degree relatives of RLS patients, as well as 85 first-degree relatives and 202 second-degree relatives of controls. The authors found that first- and second-degree relatives of RLS patients were affected with RLS significantly more often than were relatives of controls. They also found that the risk of RLS in first-degree relatives of patients with early ages of onset (i.e., onset before age 45 years) was increased 6.7-fold over that in first-degree relatives of controls. These data clearly prove a genetic etiology of RLS.

GENETICS OF FATAL FAMILIAL INSOMNIA

Fatal familial insomnia (FFI) is a rare and rapidly progressive autosomal dominant prion disease with a mutation at codon 178 of the prion protein gene (PrP). Based on biochemical, genetic, and transmission studies, it has been concluded that FFI is a transmissible prion disease resulting from a mutation at codon 178 of the PrP that is associated with the substitution of aspartic acid with asparagine, along with methionine codon present at position 129 of the mutant allele. FFI subjects are divided into homozygotes (methionine/methionine 129) and heterozygotes (methionine/valine 129). The heterozygotes pursue a longer course than the homozygotes. The same mutation at codon 178 of the prion protein gene is present in both FFI and familial Creutzfeldt-Jakob disease (CJD). These two conditions, however, are separated by the methionine-valine polymorphism at codon 129 (CJD is invariably associated with valine). FFI has been described in approximately 10 families; it has a maximum concentration in Italy but also occurs in other parts of the world. The study of FFI has begun a new era in the study of the molecular biology of the prion protein and its gene, and has once again rekindled interest in the role of the thalamus in sleep–wake regulating mechanisms.

GENETIC STUDIES OF PARASOMNIAS

Arousal disorders (nonrapid eye movement parasomnias, which include sleepwalking, sleep terrors, and confusional arousals) have been noted as having increased prevalence among family members in some studies, although their exact mode of transmission is uncertain.

Sleepwalking and sleep terrors have shown high degrees of concordance in twin studies: 50% for monozygotics; 10–15% for dizygotics. No molecular genetic studies of these arousal disorders exist.

Rapid eye movement sleep behavior disorder (RBD) exists in approximately 50% of cases, secondary to neurologic and other causes. No clear familial inheritance has been documented in idiopathic RBD, but one study showed a weak association with HLA-DQ1.

Sleep paralysis is noted not only in narcolepsy, but also as an idiopathic familial condition and occurs as physiologic sleep paralysis in individuals with normal sleep functions. In some cases, autosomal dominant transmissions have been documented. A higher concordance in monozygotic than in dizygotic twins has been documented in twin studies for sleep paralysis.

Increased familial association has been documented in some scattered reports of bruxism and head banging.

GENETIC STUDIES IN OBSTRUCTIVE SLEEP APNEA SYNDROME AND SNORING

Familial aggregates have been documented in several reports of obstructive sleep apnea syndrome. Associated risk factors, such as obesity, hypertension, alcoholism, and minor orofacial abnormalities, however, may be genetically determined, explaining the increased prevalence in other family members. Obstructive sleep apnea syndrome is multifactorial in origin; thus, genetic factors may be just one aspect of existing risks. Adequate studies, however, have not been undertaken.

Two twin studies of habitual snoring have shown higher concordance in monozygotic than in dizygotic twins.

10

Obstructive Sleep Apnea Syndrome

Obstructive sleep apnea syndrome (OSAS) is the most common sleep disorder studied by overnight polysomnographic (PSG) recording in sleep laboratories. One important study estimated that 4% of men and 2% of women between the ages of 30 and 60 years have OSAS, whereas 24% of men and 9% of women have sleep apnea (based on PSG findings of an apnea–hypopnea index [AHI] of 5, without excessive daytime somnolence [EDS]). OSAS, however, remains underdiagnosed because inadequate awareness of it, and insufficient knowledge about its serious consequences exist among physicians and the public. OSAS causes significant morbidity and mortality. Diagnosis of OSAS is important, because effective treatment for it exists. To understand this condition, certain terms related to sleep-disordered breathing must first be defined.

DEFINITION OF APNEA

The term *sleep-related apnea* refers to the temporary cessation or absence of breathing during sleep. Three types of sleep apnea have been described based on analyses of breathing patterns: upper airway obstructive, central, and mixed apneas. Cessation of airflow with no respiratory effort defines central apnea, during which both diaphragmatic and intercostal muscle activities, as well as air exchange through the nose or mouth, are absent. During upper airway obstructive sleep apnea (OSA), a cessation of airflow through the nose or mouth with persistence of the diaphragmatic and intercostal muscle activities occurs. An initial cessation of airflow with no respiratory effort (central apnea), followed by a period of upper airway OSA constitutes mixed apnea.

A few episodes of sleep apnea, particularly central apnea that occurs at the onset of nonrapid eye movement (NREM) sleep and during rapid eye movement (REM) sleep, may be noted even in individuals with normal sleep habits. To qualify as pathologic sleep apnea, apnea must last for at least 10 seconds, and the apnea index, or number of episodes of apnea per hour of sleep, must be at least 5.

DEFINITION OF HYPOPNEA

No standardized definition of hypopnea exists. Generally, however, hypopnea during sleep is defined as a decrease of airflow at the mouth and nose along with decreased respiratory effort, causing a reduction in tidal volume and amplitude of the oronasal thermistor or the pneumographic signal to half the volume measured during the preceding or following respiratory cycle. Some investigators define hypopnea as a one-third reduction of tidal volume associated with a 4% reduction of oxygen saturation.

The respiratory disturbance index (RDI), or AHI, is defined as the number of apneas plus hypopneas per hour of sleep. A normal index is less than 5. Most investigators consider AHI or RDI of 10 or more to be significant.

Apneas and hypopneas are generally accompanied by oxygen desaturation, depending on their durations, and are terminated by an arousal defined as either a transient (3–14 seconds) return of alpha activities or a change from delta to theta activities in the electroencephalogram (EEG). Repeated arousals causing sleep fragmentation are important factors that cause EDS.

DEFINITIONS OF CERTAIN OTHER TERMS USED IN SLEEP-DISORDERED BREATHING

Paradoxical breathing is characterized by movements of the thorax and abdomen in opposite directions, indicating increased upper airway resistance. Patients with OSAS and upper airway resistance syndrome (UARS) may show such breathing.

Cheyne-Stokes breathing is a type of periodic breathing characterized by cycling changes in breathing with a crescendo-decrescendo sequence separated by central apneas; the Cheyne-Stokes variant pattern of breathing is distinguished by the substitution of hypopneas for apneas. Both of these types of breathing are special types of central apneas and are most commonly noted in congestive cardiac failure and neurologic disorders.

Hypoventilation refers to the reduction of alveolar ventilation accompanied by hypoxemia and hypercapnia; it may be noted in patients with neuromuscular disorders and kyphoscoliosis.

UARS may be considered the forerunner for OSAS. In it, a general gradation occurs from an increase in the upper airway resistance found during sleep in individuals with normal sleep patterns, to loud snoring, to the stage of UARS that shows subtle partial airflow limitation, followed by complete airway occlusion (as seen in patients with OSAS). The subtle airflow limitation in UARS owing to increased upper airway resistance is followed by repeated arousals during sleep at night. Patients with UARS may or may not snore, but they do experience EDS and all its consequences (again, as seen in OSAS). The subtle airflow limitation in these patients cannot be identified using the usual respiration recording techniques (i.e., oronasal thermistor, thermocouple, inductance plethysmography, or piezoelectric strain gauge). Intraesophageal balloon manometry, however, is used to reveal increasing effort and intraesophageal pressure, leading to arousal without apnea, hypopnea, or oxygen desaturation.

EPIDEMIOLOGY OF OBSTRUCTIVE SLEEP APNEA SYNDROME

Risk of developing OSAS increases with age; there are also strong associations between OSAS, male gender, and obesity (see Chapter 8). The condition is common in men 40 years of age or older, and incidence of OSAS in women is greater after menopause. People who are overweight or obese are at increased risks for OSAS. Being "overweight" is currently defined as having a body mass index (body weight in kg divided by height in m^2) of 25 or greater; "obese" as having an index of 30 or greater. Obesity is present in approximately 70% of patients with OSAS. A strong relationship exists between neck circumference, abdominal measurement, and OSAS. Men whose necks measure more than 17 in. and women whose necks measure more than 16 in. in circumference are at risk for OSAS.

Familial aggregates of OSAS exist. Race may also be a factor, because a high prevalence of sleep-disordered breathing is seen in Pacific Islanders, Mexican-Americans, and African-Americans. Other factors highly associated with OSAS are alcohol, smoking, and drug use. Table 10.1 lists risk factors.

CONSEQUENCES OF OBSTRUCTIVE SLEEP APNEA SYNDROME

OSAS is associated with increased morbidity and mortality. Both short- and long-term consequences exist (Table 10.2). Prevalence of hypertension is noted in excess of 40% in untreated OSAS; in contrast, only 30% of patients with idiopathic hypertension have OSAS. Several inves-

Table 10.1
Risk factors for obstructive sleep apnea syndrome

Male gender
Menopausal women
Increasing age
Body mass index (≥25 is considered overweight; ≥30 is considered obese)
Increasing neck circumference (>17 in. in men; >16 in. in women)
Racial factors (increasing prevalence in Pacific Islanders, Mexican-Americans,
  and African-Americans)
Alcohol
Smoking
Increasing drug use

---

tigators noted a clear improvement of hypertension after treatment of OSAS, although a direct causal relationship has not been established. A significant relationship between hypertension and RDI has been observed, even after we eliminate obesity and other confounding factors. Repeated hypoxemias during sleep at night and increased sympathetic activity are cited as possible factors responsible for hypertension in OSAS. Cardiac arrhythmias, pulmonary hypertension, and cor pulmonale are also thought to be related to severe hypoxemias during sleep in severe cases of OSAS. Although strong relationships exist between snoring, sleep apnea, and myocardial infarction, vigorous epidemiologic studies are needed to clearly document such associations.

Table 10.2
Consequences of obstructive sleep apnea syndrome (OSAS)

Short-term consequences
  Impairment of quality of life
  Increasing traffic and work-related accidents
Long-term consequences
  Increasing prevalence of hypertension in untreated OSAS
  A strong relationship between snoring, myocardial infarction, and stroke
  Increasing association between supratentorial and infratentorial infarctions,
    transient ischemic attacks, snoring, and sleep apnea
  Neuropsychological evidence of cognitive dysfunction
  Congestive cardiac failure (cor pulmonale)
  Cardiac arrhythmias

Table 10.3
Pathogenesis of obstructive sleep apnea syndrome (OSAS)

Neural factors
    Reduced medullary respiratory neuronal output as a result of abnormal
        respiratory neural control
        Loss of tonic and phasic motor output to upper airway dilator muscle,
            causing increased upper airway resistance
Oropharyngeal anatomic factors
    Decreased tone of the upper airway dilator muscles during sleep, more
        marked during rapid eye movement sleep
        Collapse of the pharyngeal airway, causing decreased airway space
        Increased upper airway resistance
        Turbulent flow and vibration, causing snoring
        Significant narrowing or occlusion in some individuals, causing apnea
            or hypopnea
    Increased fat deposition in the region of pharynx and soft palate
        Obesity
        Myxedema
        Acromegaly
    Abnormal facial features (retrognathia, micrognathia) and unduly long or
        low-hanging uvula, causing smaller upper airway space
    Narrow upper airway space on imaging studies in many OSAS patients
    Adenotonsillar enlargement in children and craniofacial dysostosis, causing
        narrow upper airway space

PATHOGENESIS OF OBSTRUCTIVE SLEEP APNEA SYNDROME

Both local anatomic and neurologic factors play a role in the pathogenesis of OSAS (Table 10.3).

Episodes of upper airway narrowing—causing apneas, hypopneas, or increased upper airway resistance terminated by arousals and sleep fragmentation, with repetition of these cycles throughout the night—are responsible for daytime symptoms in OSAS. The site of narrowing in most cases is considered to be located at the level of the soft palate. The most important factors contributing to upper airway obstruction in OSAS (in addition to local anatomic factors) include decreased tone in the palatal, genioglossal, and other upper airway muscles, causing increased airway resistance, decreased airway space, and deposit of fatty tissue. Defective upper airway reflexes may also play a role in upper airway occlusion.

Increasing familial incidence of OSAS may be related to abnormal facial features, narrow upper airway, and long uvula, which have been found in many family members with OSAS.

As a result of abnormal neural control of medullary respiratory neurons, a marked reduction in medullary respiratory neuronal activity exists during sleep in susceptible patients. This reduction causes marked loss of tonic and phasic motor output of the upper airway dilator muscles, resulting in an increase in upper airway resistance. The chemical control of breathing is normal in OSAS, but in obesity-hypoventilation syndrome (pickwickian syndrome), which may be considered an advanced stage of OSAS in obese patients, hypoxic and hypercapnic ventilatory responses are depressed, causing hypercapnia and hypoxemia, even during wakefulness. Thus, a complex interaction of peripheral upper airway and central neural factors combine to produce the full-blown syndrome of OSAS.

SYMPTOMS OF OBSTRUCTIVE SLEEP APNEA SYNDROME

Symptoms of OSAS can be divided into two groups (Table 10.4): those occurring during sleep and those occurring during daytime hours. Major nocturnal symptoms include a long history of loud snoring and

Table 10.4
Symptoms and signs in obstructive sleep apnea syndrome

Nocturnal symptoms during sleep
    Loud snoring (often with a long history)
    Choking during sleep
    Cessation of breathing (witnessed apneas by the bed partner)
    Sitting up or fighting for breath
    Abnormal motor activities (e.g., thrashing about in bed)
    Severe sleep disruption
    Gastroesophageal reflux causing heartburn
    Nocturia and nocturnal enuresis (mostly in children)
    Insomnia (in some cases)
    Excessive nocturnal sweating (in some cases)
Daytime symptoms
    Excessive daytime somnolence
    Forgetfulness
    Personality changes
    Decreased libido and impotence in men
    Dryness of mouth on awakening
    Morning headache (in some patients)
    Automatic behavior with retrograde amnesia
    Hyperactivity (in children)
    Hearing impairment (in some patients)

Table 10.5
Physical findings in obstructive sleep apnea syndrome

Obesity (in the majority of cases)
   Increased body mass index (>25)
   Increased neck circumference (>17 in. in men and >16 in. in women)
In some patients
   Large edematous uvula
   Low-hanging soft palate
   Large tonsils and adenoids (especially in children)
   Retrognathia
   Micrognathia
   Hypertension
   Cardiac arrhythmias
   Evidence of congestive cardiac failure

---

repeated episodes of cessation of breathing (witnessed apneas by the bed partner) followed by recurrent arousals. The major daytime symptom is EDS. Patients fall asleep at inappropriate times and in inappropriate places and may be involved in driving accidents. A history of witnessed apneas by a patient's bed partner is a strong indicator of the presence of sleep apnea. Symptoms of OSAS may be aggravated by alcohol intake, central nervous system depressants, sleep deprivation, respiratory allergies, and smoking.

Physical examination should include not only general physical findings, but also an assessment of respiratory, oropharyngeal, neurologic, hematologic, and cardiovascular functions. Table 10.5 lists the pertinent physical findings that may be uncovered, including risk factors associated with repeated hypoxemia and apnea during sleep, such as hypertension, cardiac arrhythmias, and evidence of congestive cardiac failure.

LABORATORY ASSESSMENT OF OBSTRUCTIVE SLEEP APNEA SYNDROME

Laboratory investigations of OSAS must be considered extension of patient histories and physical examinations. The two most important laboratory tests for diagnosis of OSAS are overnight PSG study and Multiple Sleep Latency Test (MSLT).

Polysomnographic Study

An overnight PSG study is the single most important laboratory test used in diagnosing and treating patients with OSAS. All-night PSG (rather than a single-day nap) study is required. A single-day nap study generally misses REM sleep and its accompanying severe obstructive events and maximum oxygen desaturation. For continuous positive airway pressure (CPAP) titration, an all-night sleep study is essential. PSG study includes simultaneous recordings of various physiologic characteristics, which allows for the assessment of sleep stages and wakefulness, respiration, cardiocirculatory functions, and body movements. The standard for sleep staging is still the Rechtschaffen and Kales, technique of sleep scoring, which must be performed by manual methods, as computerized scoring is, at present, unreliable. Indications of PSG in OSAS as outlined by the American Sleep Disorders Association, now known as the American Academy of Sleep Medicine, are summarized in Chapter 4.

Characteristic PSG findings in OSAS include recurrent episodes of apneas and hypopneas, which are mostly obstructive and mixed with a few central apneas, accompanied by oxygen desaturation and followed by arousals with resumption of breathing. An AHI or RDI of 5 or less is considered normal. RDI of greater than 5–19 indicates mild OSAS, 20–49 indicates moderate OSAS, and 50 or more indicates severe OSAS. In mild OSAS, oxygen saturation may remain between 80 and 89; in moderate OSAS, oxygen saturation stays between 70 and 79; and in severe cases, oxygen saturation falls to 69 or below.

Preferably, PSG recordings should be performed in a laboratory. The American Academy of Sleep Medicine Standards of Practice Committee recommends that portable studies be performed for patients with severe clinical symptoms when standard PSG is not available or if patients cannot come to a laboratory. Although portable studies are convenient and cost effective, they have severe limitations. Concerns exist about the precision and accuracy of some portable units.

Multiple Sleep Latency Test

MSLT is a test used to document objectively excessive sleepiness. A mean sleep latency less than 5 minutes is consistent with pathologic sleepiness. In most cases of moderate to severe OSAS, MSLT shows a mean sleep latency less than 5.

Imaging Studies

In selective patients, fiberoptic endoscopy may be used to locate the site of collapse of upper airway, and cephalometric radiographs of the cranial base and facial bones may be used to assess posterior airway space or maxillomandibular deficiencies. These studies are particularly important when surgical treatment is planned. Computed tomographic scans and magnetic resonance imaging may also measure cross-sectional areas of the upper airway during wakefulness; these two studies are used mostly for research purposes.

Pulmonary Function Tests

Pulmonary function tests are performed to exclude intrinsic bronchopulmonary disease, which is a cause of sleep-disordered breathing.

Other Laboratory Tests

Appropriate tests should be performed to exclude any suspected medical disorders, particularly hypothyroidism, which may cause OSAS. These tests include blood and urinalysis, electrocardiography (ECG), Holter ECG, chest radiography, and other investigations used to rule out gastrointestinal, cardiovascular, endocrine, and renal disorders.

MANAGEMENT OF OBSTRUCTIVE SLEEP APNEA SYNDROME

Treatment of OSAS is considered under the following four headings: general measures, pharmacologic agents, mechanical devices, and surgical treatment (see Table 10.5).

General Measures

General measures (Table 10.6) include avoidance of alcohol and sedatives or hypnotics in the evening, which can aggravate sleep-disordered

Table 10.6
General and pharmacologic treatment for obstructive sleep apnea syndrome

---

General measures
    Avoid alcohol, particularly in the evening
    Avoid sedatives or hypnotics
    Reduce body weight
    Participate in an exercise program
    Avoid supine position and sleep in the lateral or prone positions if apnea
      is noted predominantly in supine position
Pharmacologic treatment (partial success in mild cases)
    Protriptyline, 5–20 mg/day
    Acetazolamide, 250–750 mg/day (for central apnea at high altitude)

---

breathing events. Other general measures include reduction of body weight in obese patients and participation in a regular exercise program. In some patients, a strong positional relationship with obstructive events limited to the supine position may exist. The patient should then be recommended to remain in lateral or prone positions.

Pharmacologic Treatment

Pharmacologic treatment has not been helpful in OSAS. Pharmacologic agents, which have been used with partial success to treat mild sleep apnea–hypopnea syndrome, include protriptyline and acetazolamide for central apnea at a high altitude (see Table 10.6).

Mechanical Devices

Perhaps the most important therapy for treating OSAS is nasal CPAP, which acts as an air splint opening up the upper airway passage so that obstructive apneas and hypopneas, hypoxemias, arousals, and sleep fragmentation are eliminated. During an overnight PSG study, after optimal CPAP pressure is determined, the patient can purchase a home unit to use nightly during sleep. The patient must use the unit every night, otherwise symptoms reappear. Some patients may require bi-level positive airway pressure, which delivers higher pressure during inspiration and lower pressure during expiration. The patient must undergo a follow-up for the purposes of compliance and to identify those patients who did not receive adequate benefit, and may therefore require repeat titration. Compliance with CPAP is approximately 70%. Reasons for noncompliance with CPAP include various adverse effects, such as difficulty with the mask, claustrophobia, air leaks occurring between mask and face, and nasal congestion (Table 10.7). Further study is needed to determine the factors responsible for compliance and noncompliance, as well as to understand long-term effects and natural histories of OSAS patients.

Dental appliances can reduce snoring and help patients control mild sleep apnea, but predicting which patients will respond to particular treatments is not possible. A tongue-retaining device is another unpredictable measure for treating sleep apnea. Table 10.8 lists mechanical devices useful in OSAS.

Surgical Treatment

In some severe cases of OSAS, CPAP therapy may fail and uvulopalatopharyngoplasty (UPP)—including laser-assisted UPP and

Table 10.7
Adverse effects associated with continuous positive airway pressure

---

Secondary to flow of air
    Chest and sinus discomfort
    Aerophagia
    Nocturnal arousals
    Sensation of suffocating
    Sensation of difficulty exhaling
    Pneumothorax, pneumomediastinum, pneumocephalus
Secondary to mask and straps
    Skin abrasion or rash
    Mask and mouth leaks causing conjunctivitis
    Claustrophobia
Nasal and other factors
    Rhinorrhea
    Nasal irritation and dryness
    Epistaxis
    Noise of the device
    Inconvenience and loss of intimacy
    Intolerance of the device by the bed partner

---

somnoplasty (radio-frequency UPP)—has been tried with variable success (Table 10.9). Improvement has been noted in up to 50% of patients, but many of these still need CPAP to eliminate residual apneas. CPAP treatment has replaced tracheostomy for treating obstructive or mixed apneas. The role and long-term effects of major surgeries for OSA remain uncertain. An overnight PSG should always be performed before performing UPP because, although it may eliminate snoring, it may not adequately relieve obstructive sleep apneas.

Table 10.8
Mechanical devices useful in obstructive sleep apnea syndrome

---

Nasal continuous positive airway pressure
Bilevel positive airway pressure
Dental appliance in some mild to moderate cases
Tongue-retaining device in mild to moderate cases (unpredictable)

Table 10.9
Surgical measures for obstructive sleep apnea syndrome

Surgical uvulopalatopharyngoplasty (UPP)
Laser-assisted UPP
Radio-frequency UPP (somnoplasty)
Major maxillofacial surgeries
Tonsillectomy and adenoidectomy (especially for children)
Tracheostomy (rarely performed)

Some patients with severe OSAS may require other surgical approaches such as maxillofacial surgeries (e.g., hyoid myotomy and suspension or mandibular osteotomy with a genioglossus muscle advancement).

11

Insomnia

DEFINITION

Insomnia is not a disease but a symptom characterized by an insufficient amount of sleep or impaired quality of sleep. General complaints of patients with insomnia include difficulty in falling asleep or maintaining sleep, resulting in nonrefreshing and nonrestorative sleep with impairment of daytime function.

CLASSIFICATION

Insomnia is classified as transient (lasting less than a week), short-term (lasting 1–3 weeks), or chronic (persisting longer than 3 weeks). Insomnia may be listed as a prominent complaint in 14 categories of the International Classification of Sleep Disorders. Insomnia can occur in intrinsic, extrinsic, and circadian rhythm sleep disorders.

EPIDEMIOLOGY

Insomnia is the most common sleep disorder affecting the population. Several surveys have confirmed that insomnia affects approximately one-third of the adult population in the United States and is a persistent problem in 10%. Prevalence of insomnia is associated with increasing age; female sex; low socioeconomic status; divorced, widowed, or separated individuals; recent stress; and depression, drug, or alcohol abuse.

CLINICAL MANIFESTATIONS

Cardinal manifestations of insomnia are listed in Chapter 7. Daytime task performance and reaction time are reportedly impaired in patients with insomnia. However, formal cognitive and motor skill tests generally do not detect any objective evidence of impairment. Nonetheless, patients reporting sleep deprivation owing to chronic insomnia are more prone to automobile accidents than those who report fatigue from other causes. Such patients also have increased risks for major depression. Some excessive risks may be related to increasing drug or alcohol abuse in these patients.

Long-term detrimental health effects owing to insomnia have not been documented. One prospective study, however, reported that an increased chance of death from cancer, stroke, or heart disease exists in persons who sleep less than 4 hours or more than 10 hours per night. However, these results have not been corroborated and may be confounded by a number of other factors.

Objective tests for sleepiness (e.g., Multiple Sleep Latency Test) generally indicate that insomniacs are less sleepy than normal control subjects, suggesting a state of hyperarousal occurs in insomnia. These findings may also result from impaired sleep perceptions. Reports indicate that more than 70% of patients with chronic insomnia (versus 30% of subjects with normal sleep habits) report being awake after awakening from stage II nonrapid eye movement sleep, and insomniacs tend to overestimate sleep latency after nocturnal awakenings.

CAUSES OF INSOMNIA

Insomnia may result from a wide variety of factors; multiple causes may contribute to it in a given individual, and different causes may be responsible for different types of insomnia.

Table 11.1 lists causes of transient and short-term insomnia. Factors resulting in transient or short-term insomnia are similar, but greater magnitudes of disturbances occur in short-term insomnia.

Jet lag is experienced after a person travels across several time zones, disrupting synchronization between the body's inner clock and its external cues. Factors detrimental to sleep include long periods of travel with limited mobility, dryness of the eyes, headache, fatigue, gastrointestinal disturbances, and nasal congestion. Symptoms are generally most pronounced when individuals travel from west to east and are more severe in the elderly than in younger individuals. Readjustment and resynchronization may occur at rates of approximately 1 hour per day when traveling eastward and 1.5 hours per day when traveling westward.

Shift work may affect up to 5 million workers in the United States and may include sleep disruption, chronic fatigue, and gastrointesti-

Table 11.1
Causes of transient or short-term insomnia

Change in sleeping environment (the most common cause of transient
     insomnia: the so-called first night effect)
Unpleasant room temperature
Excessive noise
Jet lag
Shift work
Stressful life events (e.g., loss of a loved one, divorce, loss of employment,
     preparing to take an examination)
Acute medical or surgical illnesses (including intensive care unit synrome)
Ingestion of stimulant medications (e.g., theophylline, beta blockers, cortico-
     steroids, bronchodilators, thyroxine, or withdrawal of central nervous
     system depressant medications)

---

nal symptoms (including peptic ulcer), all of which increase chances
of becoming involved in traffic accidents and making errors while on
the job.

Table 11.2 lists causes of chronic insomnia. Chronic insomnia may
result from a variety of primary sleep disorders; medical, neurologic,
or psychiatric disorders; or from chronic drug or alcohol use.

Table 11.2
Causes of chronic insomnia

Primary sleep disorders
    Idiopathic insomnia
    Psychophysiologic insomnia
    Sleep state misperception
    Inadequate sleep hygiene
    Insufficient sleep syndrome
    Restless legs syndrome
    Periodic limb movements in sleep disorder
    Circadian rhythm disorders
    Altitude insomnia
    Central sleep apnea–insomnia syndrome
General medical disorders
Neurologic disorders
Psychiatric disorders
Drug or alcohol-related insomnia

IDIOPATHIC INSOMNIA

The onset of idiopathic insomnia, which sometimes runs in families, occurs in early childhood. Patients have lifelong difficulties with initiating or maintaining sleep, or both, resulting in poor daytime functioning. Diagnosis depends on the exclusion of concomitant medical, neurologic, psychiatric, or psychological disturbances. Neurochemical imbalances that cause either hyperactivity of the arousal system or hypoactivity of sleep-promoting neurons have been suggested as contributing factors, but this idea has not been proven.

PSYCHOPHYSIOLOGIC INSOMNIA

The onset of psychophysiologic insomnia occurs during young adulthood, and symptoms may persist for decades. Psychophysiologic insomnia is a chronic insomnia with increased tension or agitation that results from learned sleep-preventing associations. Patients are over-concerned and over-focused on sleep problems, but they do not have generalized anxiety or any other psychiatric disorders. Sometimes, a family history exists, suggesting a possible genetic component is inherent.

The development of conditioned responses incompatible with sleep is the predominant feature of psychophysiologic insomnia. Insomnia is an event initiated by a stressor, but it persists even after that initial stress is gone. Factors contributing to negative conditioning and sleeplessness include excess worries; fear and frustration about being unable to initiate and maintain sleep; and the identification of the bedroom as an arousal signal. Patients generally sleep poorly during polysomnographic (PSG) study, although, occasionally, some patients sleep better because they are removed from their usual sleep environments. Patients with psychophysiologic insomnia confine anxiety to sleep-related issues, which differentiates them from patients with generalized anxiety disorders.

SLEEP STATE MISPERCEPTION

Subjective complaints of sleepiness without objective evidence (e.g., PSG evidence of insomnia) characterizes sleep state misperception. Actigraphy (which measures sleep–wake activity) or PSG recording documents normal sleep patterns in patients.

INADEQUATE SLEEP HYGIENE

Patients with inadequate sleep hygiene abuse the good "sleep hygiene measures" that promote sleep. Such sleep hygiene measures include the avoidance of caffeinated beverages, alcohol, and tobacco in the evening; avoidance of intense mental activities and vigorous exercise close to bedtime; avoidance of daytime naps and excessive time spent in bed; and adherence to a regular sleep–wake schedule.

INSUFFICIENT SLEEP SYNDROME

The most common cause of insomnia in the general population is insufficient sleep syndrome, caused by chronic sleep deprivation. Sleep deprivation results from various factors, including lifestyle, competitive drive to perform, environmental light, and sound. Daytime sleepiness, irritability, lack of concentration, decreased daytime performance, muscle aches and pains, and depression may result from chronic sleep deprivation.

ALTITUDE INSOMNIA

Altitude insomnia refers to the sleeplessness that develops in some individuals on ascent to altitudes higher than 4,000 m, occurring in conjunction with other features of acute mountain sickness (e.g., fatigue, headache, and loss of appetite). Severity of sleep disturbance is directly related to height of ascent. Individuals who live at high altitudes may become acclimatized and sleep normally, but some develop chronic mountain sickness, causing sleep disturbance. Affected individuals have Cheyne-Stokes–type periodic breathing caused by the stimulation of peripheral chemoreceptors by hypobaric hypoxemia. This process causes hyperventilation, hypocapnia, and respiratory alkalosis, which suppresses ventilation. Abnormal breathing patterns in patients tend to cause repeated awakenings with sleep fragmentation, which may be exacerbated by stress, an uncomfortable sleeping environment, and cold temperatures. The best treatment for altitude insomnia is acetazolamide, which promotes a mild metabolic acidosis, compensating for hypoxemia-driven respiratory alkalosis.

Restless legs syndrome, periodic limb movements in sleep disorder, and circadian rhythm disorders are other important causes of primary sleep disorders that result in persistent insomnia. These have been described in Chapters 13 and 17.

CENTRAL SLEEP APNEA–INSOMNIA SYNDROME

Central sleep apnea is a heterogeneous condition that may be associated with insomnia. Excessive daytime sleepiness is the most common symptom, but some patients also present with insomnia. This condition can be idiopathic or occur in association with other factors such as neuromuscular disorders, brain stem and other central neurologic lesions, left ventricular failure, and ascent to high altitudes.

GENERAL MEDICAL DISORDERS CAUSING INSOMNIA

Medical disorders that cause insomnia are listed in Table 11.3. Insomnia can also result as a side effect of medications required for treatment of general medical disorders. For example, untreated congestive cardiac failure can cause sleep disruption due to paroxysmal nocturnal dyspnea, whereas treatment with diuretics may disturb sleep via nocturia. Analogous situations may occur with nocturnal angina, chronic obstructive pulmonary disease, and bronchial asthma. Nocturnal exacerbations of asthma with cough and wheezing may be related to several circadian factors.

Table 11.3
General medical causes of insomnia

Ischemic heart disease
Nocturnal angina
Congestive cardiac failure
Chronic obstructive pulmonary disease
Bronchial asthma
Peptic ulcer disease
Gastroesophageal reflux disease
Rheumatic disorders (including fibromyalgia syndrome, rheumatoid arthritis, osteoarthritis, ankylosing spondylitis, Sjögren's syndrome)
Acquired immunodeficiency syndrome
Chronic fatigue syndrome
Lyme disease
Dermatologic disorders (e.g., nocturnal pruritus)
Systemic cancer

Table 11.4
Neurologic causes of insomnia

Brain tumors
Cerebral hemispheric and brain stem strokes
Neurodegenerative disorders (including Alzheimer's disease and Parkinson's disease)
Traumatic brain injury causing post-traumatic insomnia
Neuromuscular disorders (including painful peripheral neuropathies)
Headache syndromes (e.g., migraine, cluster and hypnic headaches and exploding head syndrome)
Fatal familial insomnia (a rare prion disease)

NEUROLOGIC DISORDERS CAUSING INSOMNIA

Structural lesions affecting the hypnogenic neurons in the preoptic-anterior hypothalamic area and the lower brain stem region in the area of the nucleus tractus solitarius can alter the balance between the waking and sleeping brain, causing insomnia. Other neurologic conditions can produce confusional episodes, changes in sensory-motor systems, pain, or movement disorders, each of which may interfere with sleep. In some neuromuscular disorders, insomnia may be caused by sleep-related hypoventilation with consequent sleep fragmentation or by medications used to treat neurologic illnesses (e.g., dopaminergic agents, anticholinergics, or anticonvulsants). Table 11.4 lists neurologic causes of insomnia.

PSYCHIATRIC DISORDERS AND INSOMNIA

Insomnia commonly coexists or precedes the development of a number of psychiatric illnesses. Surveys have shown that individuals with insomnia are more likely to develop new psychiatric disorders—particularly major depression—within 6–12 months. Anxiety disorders, depression, and schizophrenia are some of the major psychiatric disorders that may be associated with insomnia.

ASSESSMENT OF PATIENTS WITH INSOMNIA

Taking a careful history (including sleep history) is the first step in assessing insomnia patients. Sleep history should include a review of

Table 11.5
Assessment of patients with insomnia

History
    Sleep history
    Sleep diary
    Alcohol and drug history
    Psychiatric history
    Medical and neurologic history
    Family history
Physical examination
Laboratory evaluation
    Polysomnography
    Actigraphy
    Other laboratory tests to uncover neurologic or other medical conditions
        that cause insomnia

---

sleep habits, drug and alcohol consumption, medical, psychiatric, and neurologic illness, and family history (Table 11.5). An interview with the bed partner or caregiver (or, in the case of children, a parent) is important for obtaining essential information. Physical examination is used to uncover any underlying neurologic or other medical condition causing insomnia.

The entire 24-hour sleep–wake cycle, not just the events that occur at sleep onset or during the night, should be taken into consideration when evaluating sleep complaints. Specific points that should be ascertained by sleep history include the following:

- Onset of insomnia. Sudden onset suggests that a change in the sleep environment or a stressful life event may be responsible.
- Whether insomnia is transient, intermittent, or persistent. Persistent insomnia is usually a consequence of a primary sleep disorder or medical, neurologic, or psychiatric illness.
- Whether sleep complaints include initiation or maintenance problems.
- Whether the patient is preoccupied with bedtime rituals, which suggests psychological insomnia.
- Whether symptoms occur around sleep onset (e.g., paresthesia and uncomfortable limb movements occur in restless legs syndrome); during sleep (e.g., repeated awakenings, snoring, or cessation of breathing in sleep apnea syndrome); or during the day (e.g., fatigue, irritability, or lack of concentration).

- Whether the patient has frequent or early morning awakenings. Frequent awakenings are observed when insomnia occurs secondary to drugs or underlying medical conditions. Early morning awakenings frequently occur secondary to depression.
- Whether the patient has excessive daytime sleepiness.

Sleep Diary

A sleep log or diary kept for a 2-week period provides valuable information about sleep hygiene and assists in the recognition of circadian sleep disturbances. A sleep diary should capture information about bedtime, arising time, daytime naps, amount of time required to fall asleep, number of nocturnal awakenings, total sleep time, and subjective evaluation of sleep.

Alcohol and Drug History

Patients should be questioned about use of certain drugs that may directly cause insomnia and about withdrawal of central nervous system depressant drugs. Alcohol, caffeine, and tobacco consumption should be documented because they can adversely affect sleep.

Family History

A family history of insomnia may suggest certain primary sleep disorders. For example, a positive family history is found in approximately one-third of patients with idiopathic restless legs syndrome.

Physical Examination

Careful physical examination may direct attention to the presence of neurologic and other medical disorders involving the respiratory, cardiovascular, and gastrointestinal systems. Medications needed to treat such conditions may result in insomnia.

Laboratory Evaluation

Laboratory tests are not required in routine evaluations of every patient with insomnia. Two important laboratory tests that may be required in selective patients are PSG and actigraphy. The diagnosis of insomnia is primarily a clinical one, and indications for PSG in the evaluation of insomnia complaints are limited. PSG may be useful in the following situations: suspected sleep-related breathing disorder or periodic limb movements in sleep disorder; if insomnia has been present for longer than 6 months and all medical, neurologic, and psychiatric causes have been excluded; and if insomnia has not responded to behavioral or pharmacologic treatment.

Actigraphy

Actigraphy is a recently developed technique that acts as an activity monitor or motion detector to record activities during sleep and waking. Actigraphic recording conducted over several days complements sleep diaries and is useful in the diagnosis of circadian rhythm sleep disorders, sleep state misperception, and other primary types of insomnia.

Other Laboratory Tests

Neuroimaging and various other laboratory tests may be useful in diagnosing neurologic and other medical conditions that may produce insomnia.

TREATMENT OF INSOMNIA

Insomnia is a syndrome, not a specific disease; therefore, treatment is dependent on its underlying cause. Unless the primary cause of the disturbance is diagnosed and treated, treatment of secondary insomnia is unlikely to be successful.

Nonpharmacologic Treatment

Standard treatment for patients with chronic insomnia consists of nonpharmacologic measures used in conjunction with the judicious and intermittent use of hypnotics. Nonpharmacologic interventions include sleep hygiene measures, relaxation therapy (including biofeedback), stimulus control therapy, and sleep restriction treatment (Table 11.6).

Sleep Hygiene Measures

Sleep hygiene measures are listed in Table 11.7 and include simple common sense measures that address sleep habits, attitudes, and factors potentially detrimental to good sleep.

Relaxation Therapy

Relaxation therapy includes progressive muscle relaxation and biofeedback and reduces somatic arousal.

Table 11.6
Treatment of insomnia

Nonpharmacologic treatment
    Sleep hygiene measures
    Relaxation therapy (including biofeedback)
    Stimulus control therapy
    Sleep restriction therapy
Pharmacologic treatment
    Benzodiazepines
        Flurazepam, 15–30 mg
        Estazolam, 1–2 mg
        Lorazepam, 1–2 mg
        Clonazepam, 0.5–2.0 mg
        Temazepam, 15–30 mg
        Triozolam, 0.125–0.250 mg
    Nonbenzodiazepines
        Zolpidem (Ambien), 5–10 mg
        Antihistamines
        Sedative antidepressants
        Melatonin

Stimulus Control Therapy

Bootzin's stimulus control technique is directed at discouraging learned associations between bedroom and wakefulness, and re-establishing the bedroom as the major stimulus for sleep (Table 11.8). These techniques have been reported to improve insomnia complaints in approximately 50% of individuals after 1 year.

Table 11.7
Sleep hygiene measures

Restrict sleep to amount needed to feel rested.
Avoid forcing sleep.
Keep a regular sleep–wake schedule, including weekends.
Avoid caffeinated beverages after lunch.
Avoid alcohol near bedtime (i.e., no "night cap").
Avoid smoking, especially in the evening.
Do not go to bed hungry.
Adjust bedroom environment.
Exercise regularly for at least 20 mins, preferably 4–5 hrs before bedtime.
Do not engage in planning next day's activities at bedtime.

Table 11.8
Stimulus control treatment

Go to bed only when sleepy.
Do not watch television, read, eat, or worry while in bed.
Use bed only for sleep and intimacy.
Get out of bed if unable to fall asleep in 15–20 mins and go to another room.
  Return to bed only when sleepy. Repeat this step as many times as necessary throughout the night.
Set alarm clock to wake up at a fixed time each morning (including weekends).
Do not take a nap during the day.

Sleep Restriction Therapy

Restricting total sleep time in bed may improve sleep efficiency. Later, gradually increasing allotted sleep time may improve level of daytime function and overall sleep quality. Approximately one-fourth of patients with insomnia benefit from such a regimen.

The best nonpharmacologic approach has not been established. In one meta-analysis involving 2,102 patients in 59 trials, sleep restriction and stimulus control therapies were found to be more effective than relaxation techniques when used alone. Sleep hygiene measures did not show evidence of efficacy. The extent to which concomitant use of nonpharmacologic therapy augments the performance of pharmacologic treatment is also unclear. Both nonpharmacologic and pharmacologic therapies may be useful in the management of insomnia. One randomized study of 78 patients with insomnia used three methods of therapy to treat insomnia: cognitive-behavioral therapy, including sleep restriction and stimulus control treatment; pharmacotherapy with temazepam; and a combination of pharmacologic and nonpharmacologic therapies. These three active treatment measures had better results than did the placebo after 3 months. Cognitive-behavioral therapy was associated with most sustained improvement in sleep over a 24-month follow-up period.

Pharmacologic Treatment

Hypnotic agents may be helpful in treating transient or short-term insomnia; however, their use should be restricted to less than 4 weeks' duration. Intermittent use of hypnotics (e.g., 1–2 nights per week) may be necessary in some patients with chronic insomnia who do not respond adequately to nonpharmacologic treatment, although drugs should not be the major component of therapy.

Hypnotic medications are contraindicated in pregnancy, because an increased risk of fetal malformation exists when diazepam or chlordiazepoxide is used during the first trimester. Drugs should also be avoided or used cautiously in patients with alcoholism or renal, hepatic, or pulmonary disease. A combination of alcohol and hypnotics is absolutely contraindicated. Hypnotic drugs also should be avoided in patients with sleep apnea syndrome.

Benzodiazepine Hypnotics

Four benzodiazepine drugs are commonly used as hypnotics in the United States: temazepam, flurazepam, estazolam, and triazolam. Two other benzodiazepine drugs, lorazepam and clonazepam, also are used frequently for this indication. Triazolam is no longer available in Great Britain because serious side effects, such as amnesia, rebound insomnia, and anxiety, have been reported. It is used cautiously in the United States.

Benzodiazepine's mechanism of action in treating insomnia is not quite clear. Benzodiazepine often produces subjective improvement without an appreciable objective improvement in PSG studies. Selection of specific hypnotic agents depends on the elimination half-life. Short-acting drugs, such as temazepam, estazolam, and triazolam, are generally preferable because they produce less residual sleepiness the morning after use. These drugs may, however, have a high incidence of amnesia and rebound insomnia and should be used cautiously in patients with anxiety disorders. In elderly patients or those with renal and hepatic dysfunction, doses may be adjusted due to prolonged elimination half-life. Dependence and tolerance are major disadvantages long-term hypnotic use. These drugs should be discontinued gradually rather than abruptly to avoid precipitating symptoms of withdrawal.

Nonbenzodiazepine Hypnotics

Zolpidem is a nonbenzodiazepine hypnotic used in the short-term treatment of insomnia. This drug activates the benzodiazepine receptor, but it does not have a benzodiazepine structure. Similar to benzodiazepine, zolpidem produces improvement in sleep perception rather than objective evidence in PSG study. Zolpidem is a short-acting drug and produces less residual somnolence than benzodiazepine hypnotics.

A number of sedating antidepressants (e.g., amitriptyline and trazodone) have been used in the management of patients with depression and insomnia; they have limited usefulness in nondepressed patients, who rapidly develop tolerances to sedative effects.

Many over-the-counter sleep medications contain the sedating antihistamines diphenhydramine or doxylamine. These drugs have half-lives of 8.5–10.0 hours and may, therefore, result in decreased alertness, daytime sedation, and prolonged reaction time on the day after their use. Dizziness, dryness of the mouth, constipation, and blurring of vision also may occur. These medications are generally not helpful in the management of chronic insomnia.

Melatonin, a normal product of the pineal gland, is sold as a food supplement and an orphan drug in the United States, but over-the-counter sales of melatonin in the United Kingdom are banned. The drug is generally used to correct circadian rhythm sleep disorders in blind persons with no light perception. Sometimes it has been useful in treating jet lag and delayed sleep phase syndrome, but the hormone does not appear to be a potent hypnotic for most patients with chronic insomnia. Furthermore, data regarding the efficacy and safety of melatonin are minimal. A subgroup of elderly patients with low melatonin levels, however, have benefited from melatonin treatment.

The treatment of insomnia owing to restless legs syndrome and periodic limb movements in sleep disorder is addressed in Chapter 13.

12

Narcolepsy and Idiopathic Hypersomnia

The term *narcolepsy* was coined in 1880 by the French physician Gellinau, who gave a classic description of irresistible sleep attacks in patients and described all clinical features of cataplexy under the heading of "astasia." Reports of a large series of narcoleptic patients in the twentieth century brought narcolepsy to the forefront of the medical profession. Sleep attacks, cataplexy, sleep paralysis, and hypnagogic hallucinations were all grouped under the term *narcoleptic tetrad* by Yoss and Daly in 1957. In 1960, Vogel discovered sleep onset rapid eye movements (SOREMs). Finally, the discovery of the presence of HLA-DR2 and DQw1 (now called *DQw15*) antigens in 100% of Japanese narcoleptic patients by Honda et al. brought narcolepsy research to the forefront of the molecular neurobiology field.

EPIDEMIOLOGY AND GENETICS OF NARCOLEPSY

The prevalence of narcolepsy is estimated to be 3–6 per 10,000 people in the United States, 1 person per 600 in Japan, and 1 in 500,000 people in Israel; a distinct lack of good epidemiologic study in different parts of the world exists. The genetics of narcolepsy have been described in Chapter 9.

CLINICAL MANIFESTATIONS

In most cases, the onset of narcolepsy occurs in adolescents or young adults who experience excessive daytime somnolence (EDS) and sleep attacks; it is a lifelong condition. Peak incidences mostly occur between the ages of 15 and 20 years. A second peak is observed after the second

Table 12.1
Clinical manifestations of narcolepsy

Major manifestations
    Narcoleptic sleep attacks: 100%
    Cataplexy: 70%
    Sleep paralysis: 25–50%
    Hypnagogic hallucinations: 20–40%
    Disturbed night sleep: 70–80%
    Automatic behavior: 20–40%
Associated features
    Sleep apnea
    Periodic limb movements in sleep
    Rapid eye movement sleep behavior disorder

---

decade of life. Rare cases have been described in children younger than 5 years and in adults older than 50 years, however. Men and women are equally affected by narcolepsy and cataplexy. At least 70% of patients develop cataplexy after a variable interval of months to years, followed by other symptoms in a smaller percentage of cases. Sometimes, cataplexy precedes EDS. Rarely do any of the other major symptoms manifest themselves before narcoleptic sleep attacks and cataplexy occur.

The clinical manifestations of narcolepsy are grouped into two broad categories, major and associated features (Table 12.1). Major manifestations include narcoleptic sleep attacks, cataplexy, sleep paralysis, hypnagogic hallucinations, disturbed night sleep, and automatic behavior.

Narcoleptic Sleep Attacks

Narcoleptic patients manifest an irresistible and uncontrollable desire to fall asleep under inappropriate circumstances and in inappropriate places (e.g., while driving, talking, eating, playing, walking, running, working, sitting, listening to lectures, or watching television or movies; during sexual intercourse; or when involved in boring or monotonous circumstances). These are brief attacks that last from a few minutes to 15–30 minutes. Patients generally feel refreshed on awakening, although they occasionally may feel tired and drowsy. A wide variation in the frequency of attacks exists; one or more attacks may occur daily, weekly, monthly, or every few weeks to months, or they may occur occasionally (e.g., once every year or few years). Attacks persist throughout a patient's lifetime, although fluctuations and rare temporary remissions may occur. Patients may show declines in performance at school and work and encounter psychosocial and socioeconomic difficulties as a result of sleep attacks and EDS.

Cataplexy

Cataplexy is characterized by a sudden loss of tone in all voluntary muscles except respiratory and ocular muscles. More than 95% of the time, attacks are triggered by emotional factors such as laughter, rage, or anger. Attacks may be complete or partial and are rarely unilateral. Patients completely lose tone in limb muscles and fall to the ground. Buckling of the knees, nodding of the head, sagging of the jaws, dysarthria, or loss of voice may occur. Attacks generally last for a few seconds to a minute; sometimes they last a few minutes. Consciousness is retained completely during attacks. Neurologic examination during these brief spells reveals flaccidity of the muscles and absent or markedly reduced muscle stretch reflexes. H-reflex, the electrical counterpart of the muscle stretch reflexes, and F responses are decreased or absent. Cataplexy is present in 60–100% of patients with narcolepsy. Generally, cataplexy occurs months to years after the onset of sleep attacks, but occasionally it may be the initial manifestation. Attacks often occur frequently in the beginning but may decrease in frequency later (and may disappear in old age). Rarely, *status cataplecticus* occurs, particularly after a withdrawal of tricyclic medications. During brief cataplectic spells, electroencephalogram (EEG) shows wakefulness; however, if attacks last longer than 1–2 minutes, the EEG shows rapid eye movement (REM) sleep.

Sleep Paralysis

Sleep paralysis is seen in approximately 25–50% of patients, generally months to years after the onset of narcoleptic sleep attacks. A sudden paralysis of one or both sides of the body or one limb occurs, either during sleep onset at night (hypnagogic) or on awakening (hypnopompic) in the morning. The patient is unable to move or speak and is often frightened or fearful, although he or she retains consciousness.

Hypnagogic Hallucination

Hypnagogic hallucinations occur either during the onset of sleep or on awakening in the morning and are noted in 20–40% of narcolepsy patients, generally beginning years after the onset of sleep attacks. Most commonly, these hallucinations are characterized by vivid and often fearful visual hallucinations; sometimes, however, auditory, vestibular, or somesthetic phenomena occur. In 30% of cases, three of the four major manifestations of the narcoleptic tetrad are seen; in approximately 10% of cases, all four major features occur together.

Disturbed Night Sleep

Disturbed night sleep is a major manifestation, noted in 70–80% of patients.

Automatic Behavior

Automatic behavior is observed in 20–40% of patients. During this episode, the patient repeatedly continues to perform a single function, speaks or writes in a meaningless manner, or drives on the wrong side of the road or to a strange place, then does not recall the episode. This behavior resembles a fuguelike state and may result from partial sleep episodes, frequent lapses, or "microsleeps."

ASSOCIATED FEATURES OF NARCOLEPSY

Patients with narcolepsy may also have sleep apnea, periodic limb movements in sleep (PLMS), or REM sleep behavior disorder (RBD). Sleep apnea is present in approximately 30% of narcoleptic patients and occurs most commonly as a central apnea, but also occurs as obstructive or mixed apneas. Associated sleep apnea may aggravate sleep attacks. Recognizing obstructive sleep apnea in patients is important, because patients may require additional treatment with continuous positive airway pressure (CPAP) for relief of apneas and EDS. RBD generally occurs in men with narcolepsy. Narcolepsy and RBD most commonly emerge in tandem. Treatment of narcolepsy–cataplexy with stimulants and tricyclic medications may induce or exacerbate RBD.

DIFFERENTIAL DIAGNOSIS

Conditions that should be differentiated from narcoleptic sleep attacks are listed in Table 12.2. All causes of EDS should be excluded, includ-

Table 12.2
Differential diagnosis of narcoleptic sleep attacks

Obstructive sleep apnea syndrome
Sleep deprivation
Insufficient sleep syndrome
Alcohol- and drug-related hypersomnolence
Periodic hypersomnolence
Medical, neurologic, and psychiatric disorders causing hypersomnolence
Idiopathic hypersomnia
Circadian rhythm sleep disorders

---

ing sleep deprivation; insufficient sleep syndrome; obstructive sleep apnea syndrome; alcohol- and drug-related hypersomnolence; periodic hypersomnolence; medical, neurologic, and psychiatric disorders causing hypersomnolence; idiopathic hypersomnia; and circadian rhythm sleep disorders.

Obstructive sleep apnea syndrome (OSAS), the most common cause of EDS referred to sleep laboratories for evaluation, is characterized by recurrent episodes of obstructive and mixed apneas during nonrapid eye movement (NREM) and REM sleep in overnight polysomnographic (PSG) recordings. Patients experience prolonged sleep episodes during the daytime followed by fatigue and drowsiness on awakening (in contrast to narcoleptic patients, who often experience feelings of refreshment on awakening from brief sleep attacks). A careful history and physical examination followed by an overnight PSG recording exclude all causes of hypersomnolence from narcoleptic sleep attacks.

Idiopathic hypersomnia closely resembles narcolepsy syndrome and is described in the section Idiopathic Hypersomnia.

Cataplexy may be mistaken for partial complex seizures, absence spells, atonic seizures, drop attacks, and syncope. A partial complex seizure is characterized by an altered state of consciousness, unlike cataplexy, in which consciousness is retained. In addition, patients with partial complex seizures may have generalized tonic-clonic movements, postictal confusion, and may show epileptiform discharges in the anterior and mediotemporal regions in the EEG.

Absence spells are characterized by staring, vacant expressions lasting for a few seconds to 30 seconds and altered states of alertness that are associated with characteristic 3-Hz spike and wave discharges in EEG.

Atonic seizures are accompanied by transient losses of consciousness and EEG evidence of slow spike and wave or polyspike and wave discharges.

Drop attacks may occur in vertebrobasilar insufficiency (transient ischemic attacks); patients may exhibit other evidence of brain stem ischemia, such as vertigo, ataxia, or diplopia. Syncope (transient loss of consciousness) may result from cardiogenic or other causes, including neurogenic orthostatic hypotension.

Narcoleptic sleep paralysis should be differentiated from isolated, physiologic, and familial sleep paralysis. In all of these conditions, other manifestations of narcolepsy are absent.

Automatic behavior should be differentiated from the automatism observed in partial complex seizure and psychogenic fugue. History, physical examination, and EEG should be helpful in making this differentiation.

Symptomatic or secondary narcolepsy–cataplexy may rarely be associated with diencephalic and midbrain tumors and multiple sclerosis, and should be differentiated from idiopathic narcolepsy–cataplexy syndrome.

PATHOGENESIS OF NARCOLEPSY–CATAPLEXY SYNDROME

Physiologic, neurochemical, genetic, and environmental factors all play distinct roles in the pathogenesis of narcolepsy–cataplexy syndrome (Table 12.3).

Physiologic Mechanisms

A disturbance in REM–NREM sleep–wake state boundaries is the fundamental physiologic abnormality that occurs in narcolepsy syndrome. A hallmark of physiologic testing in narcolepsy is the presence of SOREM—that is, the onset of REM sleep at (or within 15 minutes of) sleep onset. Other features also point to dissociation of REM sleep or intrusion into wakefulness. Cataplexy is characterized by wakeful EEG associated with muscle atonia of REM sleep without other features. If episodes are prolonged, patients develop full REM sleep.

In sleep paralysis, muscle atonia is similar to REM sleep atonia. During hypnagogic hallucinations, an intrusion of REM sleep with dream imagery but without other features of REM sleep occurs. In many of these episodes, the sleep state is intermediate, between REM and NREM. Many patients also experience "microsleeps," brief episodes of NREM sleep lasting 3–14 seconds, during the daytime. Total 24-hour sleep and REM sleep percentages are normal in narcoleptic patients, but the intrusion of REM sleep atonia into wakefulness suggests that a dissociation of REM sleep

Table 12.3
Pathogenesis of narcolepsy–cataplexy syndrome

Physiologic mechanisms
  Disturbed rapid eye movement (REM)–nonrapid eye movement (NREM)
    state boundary
  Presence of sleep onset REMs
  Muscle atonia of REM with awake electroencephalography but without
    other features of REM sleep as in cataplexy and sleep paralysis
  REM sleep dream imagery without other features of REM as in hypna-
    gogic hallucinations; sleep is intermediate between REM and
    NREM
  REM sleep behavior disorder in some narcoleptics
Neurochemical mechanisms
  An imbalance of cholinergic catecholaminergic regulation of REM sleep
    Muscarinic cholinergic supersensitivity
      Physostigmine (cholinergic drug) injection increases cataplectic
        episodes
      Atropine and scopolamine (muscarinic-blocking agents) decrease
        cataplectic spells
      M2 subtypes of muscarinic receptors: upregulated in pons in narco-
        leptic dogs
      M1 muscarinic receptor binding in basal ganglia and amygdala:
        increased (autopsy)
    Defective monoaminergic regulation of REM sleep
      Monoamines (norepinephrine, serotonin) play a permissive role by
        modulating cholinergic activity in REM sleep
      Increased availability of synaptic monoamines (e.g., stimulants and
        antidepressants used to treat narcolepsy-cataplexy) benefit nar-
        coleptic sleep attacks and cataplexy
      α_2-Agonists or α_1-antagonists exacerbate, whereas α_2-antagonists
        reduce cataplexy
      Cerebrospinal fluid dopamine and its metabolite homovanillic acid
        are decreased in human narcolepsy, suggesting an impaired
        dopamine release or its increased turnover

---

regulation occurs. Some narcoleptic patients manifest RBD occasionally, evidence that supports the impaired state boundary theory in narcolepsy. Based on time-isolation laboratory experiments, strong evidence for the circadian disorganization of narcoleptic patients also exists.

Neurochemical Mechanisms

The primary neurochemical defect in narcolepsy is unknown. However, evidence of an imbalance in chemical regulation between cholinergic and catecholaminergic neurons, interfering with REM sleep regulatory mechanisms within the brain stem, exists. Small doses of cholinergic drug injection (e.g., physostigmine) increase cataplectic episodes in narcoleptic dogs (e.g., Doberman pinschers) but not in control non-narcoleptic dogs, whereas atropine and scopolamine (muscarinic-blocking agents) decrease cataplectic episodes. In addition, M2 subtypes of muscarinic cholinergic receptors are reported to be upregulated in the pontine reticular formation of narcoleptic dogs. Postmortem studies have also reported an increase in muscarinic M1 receptor binding in the basal ganglia and in amygdala. These findings suggest that muscarinic cholinergic systems in cataplectic dog brains are supersensitive.

Evidence also exists to suggest a defect in monoaminergic regulation of REM sleep mechanism contributing to narcoleptic symptoms. "REM-off" cells (serotonergic cells in the raphe and noradrenergic cells in the locus ceruleus) are completely inactive during REM sleep and appear to play permissive roles by modulating cholinergic activity. Stimulants (amphetamine and others) used for effective treatment of sleepiness in narcolepsy increase the synaptic availability of norepinephrine. Tricyclic antidepressants used in the treatment of cataplexy decrease reuptake of norepinephrine, and fluoxetine (used also in cataplexy) decreases reuptake of serotonin (thus, increasing the availability of these monoamines). Prazosin, an α_1-receptor antagonist, and α_2-receptor agonists exacerbate cataplexy, whereas α_2 antagonists (e.g., yohimbine) reduce symptoms of cataplexy. These findings are consistent with the suggestion that norepinephrine and serotonin play inhibitory roles in controlling cataplexy. Cerebrospinal fluid dopamine and the dopamine metabolite homovanillic acid are decreased in human narcolepsy. Additionally, human autopsy brain samples reveal an increase of striatal dopamine D2 receptors, although these findings have been contradicted by positron emission tomography (PET) reports. These findings suggest an impairment of dopamine release or an increase in turnover. Some evidence suggests that an alteration of α-adrenergic receptors in certain brain regions exists.

Genetic and Environmental Factors

Genetic factors have been described in Chapter 9. The exact environmental factors affecting narcolepsy are unknown. Speculation about the question of autoimmunity in narcolepsy exists, but no definite evidence has been uncovered.

IDIOPATHIC HYPERSOMNIA

Idiopathic hypersomnia is a disorder of excessive sleepiness presumed (but not proven) to be caused by the central nervous system; it is associated with normal or prolonged (1–2 hours) NREM sleep episodes during the daytime. The condition occurs insidiously generally between the ages of 15 and 30 years, and it closely resembles narcolepsy. The sleep pattern in idiopathic hypersomnia is different than that in narcolepsy. The patient generally sleeps for hours, and the sleep is not refreshing. Because of excessive daytime somnolence, the condition may also be mistaken for sleep apnea. The patient, however, does not give a history of cataplexy, snoring, or repeated awakenings throughout the night. Some patients may have automatic behavior with amnesia for the events. Physical examination uncovers no abnormal neurologic findings. This is a disabling and life-long condition.

The differential diagnosis of idiopathic hypersomnia should include other causes of excessive daytime somnolence, such as narcolepsy–cataplexy, upper airway OSAS, central sleep apnea syndrome, upper airway resistance syndrome, insufficient sleep, drug-induced hypersomnia, and other medical or psychiatric disorders, particularly mood disorders (see Chapter 7). Other conditions that should be included in the differential diagnosis include post-traumatic hypersomnia, chronic fatigue syndrome, delayed sleep phase syndrome, and long sleeper syndrome. Unlike narcolepsy, no clear association exists between idiopathic hypersomnia and HLAs.

LABORATORY ASSESSMENT OF NARCOLEPSY–CATAPLEXY AND IDIOPATHIC HYPERSOMNIA

The two most important laboratory tests for the assessment of narcolepsy–cataplexy and idiopathic hypersomnia are overnight PSG study followed by Multiple Sleep Latency Test (MSLT) the next day.

Overnight PSG findings in patients with narcolepsy–cataplexy include short sleep latency, excessive disruption of sleep with frequent arousals, reduced total sleep time, excessive body movements, reduced slow wave sleep, and SOREM, noted in approximately 40–50% of cases. Some narcoleptic patients may experience associated sleep apnea, particularly central apneas, PLMS, and RBD.

In idiopathic hypersomnia, overnight PSG shows sleep with normal sleep stages and sleep cycling. In some patients, slow wave sleep may increase. Sleep apnea, PLMS, and RBD have not been observed in idiopathic hypersomnia.

MSLT is an important test to document objectively excessive sleepiness. A mean sleep latency of less than 5 minutes is consistent with pathologic sleepiness. SOREM in two or more of the four to five recordings made during MSLT is suggestive of narcolepsy, although abnormalities of REM sleep regulatory mechanism and circadian rhythm sleep disturbances also may lead to such findings. In idiopathic hypersomnia, MSLT shows pathologic sleepiness without any SOREMs.

Maintenance of Wakefulness Test (MWT) is a variant of MSLT and measures a patient's ability to stay awake. MWT is performed at 2-hour intervals in a quiet, dark room with the patient instructed to resist sleep in a semireclining position in a chair. Four or five tests are performed, each one lasting 20–40 minutes. MWT is important for monitoring the effect of treatment in narcolepsy, but it is not as good as MSLT for measuring daytime sleepiness.

HLA typing is another test that may be performed. Most narcoleptic patients are positive for HLA-DR2, DQ1, and DQB1*0602. This test, however, is not diagnostic of narcolepsy because of the high prevalence of these HLAs that occur in the non-narcoleptic population and reports of HLA-negative narcoleptics that exist.

TREATMENT OF NARCOLEPSY–CATAPLEXY SYNDROME

Administration of stimulants is the treatment of choice for narcoleptic sleep attacks (Table 12.4). In 65–85% of patients, a significant improvement of EDS can be obtained. Stimulant drugs include pemoline, methylphenidate, dextroamphetamine, methamphetamine, and, recently, Modafinil.

Methylphenidate is the drug most commonly used. In patients with mild sleepiness, however, an initial treatment with pemoline, starting with 18.75–37.50 mg in the morning, may be tried. Methylphenidate treatment may be started with 5 mg administered two to three times per day. To avoid insomnia, the last dose should not be taken after 4:00 PM. In those patients who do not respond to methylphenidate, treatment with dextroamphetamine (starting with 5–10 mg once or twice a day) can be administered. Maximum acceptable doses include, for pemoline, 150 mg per day; 50 mg per day (rarely, 100 mg) for methylphenidate; and 50 mg per day for both dextroamphetamine and methamphetamine. The most common side effects of these stimulants

Table 12.4
Drug treatment of narcolepsy

For sleep attacks
    Pemoline (Cylert): 18.75–37.50 mg/day, up to 150 mg/day
    Methylphenidate (Ritalin): 5 mg BID, 30 mins before meals, to a maximum
       of 50 mg/day (rarely, 100 mg/day)
    Dextroamphetamine (Dexedrine): 5 mg daily or BID, up to 50 mg/day
    Methamphetamine (Methedrine): 5 mg daily or BID, up to 50 mg/day
    Mazindol: 2 mg daily or BID, up to 8 mg/day
    Modafinil: 200 mg/day
For cataplexy, sleep paralysis, and hypnagogic hallucinations
    Imipramine: 75–150 mg/day
    Clomipramine: 75–125 mg/day
    Fluoxetine: 20 mg daily, up to 80 mg/day
    Viloxazine: 150–200 mg/day

include nervousness, tremor, insomnia, irritability, palpitation, headache, and gastrointestinal symptoms. Tolerance is another problem that is noted in up to 30% of patients, particularly with increasing doses.

Modafinil, a novel wake-promoting agent, has been shown to be an effective treatment for EDS associated with narcolepsy after double-blind placebo controlled trials in the United States. The dose of this medication is 200 mg in the morning, 1 hour before or after breakfast. The most common adverse effects of Modafinil include headache, nausea, nervousness, anxiety, and insomnia. Modafinil may interact with drugs that inhibit, induce, or are metabolized by cytochrome P450 enzymes such as diphenylhydantoin, diazepam, and propranolol.

Treatment of cataplexy and other auxiliary symptoms of narcolepsy (see Table 12.4) consists of the administration of tricyclic antidepressants such as protriptyline, beginning with 5 mg per day; imipramine (25–200 mg per day); and clomipramine (10–200 mg per day). Specific serotonin reuptake inhibitors such as fluoxetine, beginning with 20 mg in the morning, (which may be increased gradually to 80 mg per day), has been used with success.

Nonpharmacologic treatment of narcolepsy includes general sleep hygiene measures, short daytime naps, and narcolepsy support groups.

TREATMENT OF IDIOPATHIC HYPERSOMNIA

Treatment of idiopathic hypersomnia is similar to stimulant treatment for narcolepsy, but is unsatisfactory.

13

Motor Functions and Dysfunctions of Sleep

CHANGES IN MOTOR SYSTEMS DURING SLEEP

Considerable modulation of motor mechanisms during sleep occurs. Generally, sleep is dominated by a central inhibitory mechanism, but the excitatory mechanism intermittently breaks through the inhibitory phase in individuals with normal sleep functions, giving rise to physiologic motor activities during sleep, such as body movements, postural shifts, and hypnic jerks. Motor activity, including muscle tone, progressively decreases during nonrapid eye movement (NREM) stages I to IV sleep, with further decrement of motor activity and marked diminution or absence of muscle tone in rapid eye movement (REM) sleep (Table 13.1). When this delicate balance between inhibitory and excitatory mechanisms breaks down, pathologic or abnormal motor activities emerge during sleep. Polysomnographic (PSG) study has revealed that movements are most common during transitions to wake or lighter stages of sleep, followed by stage I NREM or REM sleep and stage II NREM sleep. During NREM stages III and IV (slow wave sleep [SWS]), no movements are noted.

Physiologic studies of motor neurons during different stages of sleep reveal that they are slightly hyperpolarized during relaxation and NREM sleep. Further hyperpolarization occurs during REM sleep due to increased frequency of inhibitory postsynaptic potentials. During REM sleep, however, bursts of myoclonic movements occur as a result of superimposed phasic excitation that results from excitatory postsynaptic potentials. Profound changes occur in the monosynaptic and polysynaptic reflexes, which are diminished during NREM sleep and almost completely abolished in REM sleep. This reduced reflex gain, which has profound clinical implications, most likely results from inhibition of motor output. Sleep-related decrement in the excitability of upper airway motor neurons causes an impairment of upper airway

Table 13.1
Changes in motor systems during sleep–wakefulness

States of Awareness	Muscle Tone	Body Movements
Wakefulness	+++++	Present
Stage I NREM	++++	Postural shifts
Stage II NREM	+++	Postural shifts
Stage III NREM	++	Relatively immobile
Stage IV NREM	+	Relatively immobile
REM	+ to –	Myoclonic bursts

+++++ to + = progressive decrement of muscle tone; – = absence of muscle tone;
NREM = nonrapid eye movement; REM = rapid eye movement.

reflex response triggered by negative intrathoracic pressure at the onset of inspiration; this impaired response makes the upper airway susceptible to suction collapse and obstructive apneas.

MOVEMENT DISORDERS AND SLEEP

Movement disorders specialists see patients with various involuntary movements that occur during the daytime, whereas sleep specialists are often consulted by patients with paroxysmal involuntary movements, abnormal posture, and behavior that occur during sleep at night. These daytime and nighttime movement disorders are quite distinct from each other. Some abnormal movements are triggered by sleep or occur preferentially during sleep, for example, whereas certain involuntary movements seen during the daytime may persist during sleep at night.

Movement disorders occurring during sleep can be classified into physiologic and pathologic types (Table 13.2). Physiologic motor activity during sleep includes postural shifts; body and limb movements; physiologic fragmentary myoclonus, consisting of phasic muscle bursts (seen typically in REM sleep); and hypnic jerks, consisting of sudden muscle jerks involving either the whole body or part of it at sleep onset during the transition between wakefulness and sleep.

Abnormal Movements during Sleep

Abnormal movements that occur during sleep consist of motor parasomnias, restless legs syndrome (RLS)–periodic limb movements in

Table 13.2
Classification of disorders of movements during sleep

I. Physiologic (normal) motor activity during sleep
  A. Postural shifts, body and limb movements during sleep
  B. Physiologic fragmentary myoclonus
  C. Hypnic jerks (sleep starts)
  D. Hypnagogic imagery
II. Pathologic (abnormal) motor activity during sleep
  A. Motor parasomnias
    1. Sleep–wake transition disorders
      a. Rhythmic movement disorder
      b. Sleep talking (somniloquy)
      c. Nocturnal leg cramps
      d. Propriospinal myoclonus at the transition from wakefulness to
        drowsiness
    2. NREM sleep parasomnias
      a. Confusional arousals
      b. Sleepwalking
      c. Sleep terror
    3. REM sleep parasomnias
      a. Nightmares
      b. REM sleep behavior disorder
    4. Diffuse parasomnias (no stage preference)
      a. Bruxism
      b. Neonatal sleep myoclonus
  B. Nocturnal seizures
    1. True nocturnal seizures
      a. Tonic seizure
      b. Benign rolandic seizure
      c. Autosomal dominant nocturnal frontal lobe seizure
      d. Nocturnal paroxysmal dystonia
      e. Paroxysmal arousals and awakening
      f. Episodic nocturnal wanderings
      g. Electrical status epilepticus in sleep
    2. True nocturnal and diurnal seizures (diffuse seizures)
      a. Generalized tonic-clonic seizure
      b. Myoclonic seizure
      c. Infantile spasms (West's syndrome)
      d. Partial complex seizure
      e. Frontal lobe seizure
      f. Epilepsia partialis continua
    3. Pseudoseizure (nonepileptic or psychogenic seizure)
  C. Involuntary movement disorders
    1. Always persisting during sleep: palatal myoclonus or palatal tremor
    2. Frequently persisting during sleep
      a. Spinal and propriospinal myoclonus
      b. Tics in Tourette's syndrome
      c. Hemifacial spasms
      d. Hyperekplexia or exaggerated startle syndrome

Table 13.2
Continued

3. Sometimes persisting during sleep
   a. Tremor
   b. Chorea
   c. Dystonia
   d. Hemiballisms
D. Drug-induced nocturnal dyskinesias
   1. Levodopa-induced myoclonus in Parkinson's disease
   2. Medication-induced (e.g., tricyclic antidepressants, levodopa, lithium) periodic limb movements
E. Periodic limb movements in sleep disorder
F. Nocturnal jerks and body movements in obstructive sleep apnea syndrome
G. Excessive fragmentary myoclonus seen in a variety of sleep disorders
H. Sleep-related panic attacks
I. Dissociative disorders

NREM = nonrapid eye movement; REM = rapid eye movement.

sleep (PLMS), nocturnal seizures, diurnal involuntary movements persisting during sleep, drug-induced nocturnal dyskinesias, jerks and body movements seen in patients with obstructive sleep apnea syndrome (OSAS), excessive fragmentary myoclonus during NREM and REM sleep seen in a variety of sleep disorders, and hyperekplexia or exaggerated startle syndrome. Several of these abnormal nocturnal movements have been described in Chapters 14 and 18. In addition, prominent sleep dysfunction has been described in specific movement disorders such as Parkinson's disease (PD) and other extrapyramidal disorders, as well as in RLS–PLMS. These sleep disturbances are briefly reviewed, and approaches for treating patients who experience movement disorders during sleep and for management of sleep dysfunction in PD and RLS–PLMS are discussed.

Parkinson's Disease and Sleep

The characteristic clinical tetrad of idiopathic PD consists of tremor at repose, rigidity, bradykinesia (slowness of voluntary movement) or akinesia (reduced or absent spontaneous movement), and a loss of postural reflexes. The pathologic hallmark of PD is the presence of Lewy bodies (intracytoplasmic eosinophilic inclusions) as well as the loss of neurons with depigmentation in the substantia nigra pars compacta (Table 13.3).

Table 13.3
Salient clinical features of Parkinson's disease

Rest tremor
Cogwheel or lead-pipe rigidity
Bradykinesia or akinesia
Loss of postural reflexes and postural impairment
Others
    Depression
    Dementia
    Dysautonomia
    Sleep disturbances

Sleep difficulties are common in PD, noted in 70–90% of patients. Sleep complaints in PD include insomnia, hypersomnia, parasomnia (abnormal movements or behavior during sleep), and circadian rhythm sleep disorders (Table 13.4).

Sleep dysfunction in PD is discussed under four broad categories: effect of PD on sleep, effect of sleep on PD, effect of antiparkinsonian drugs on sleep, and associated conditions causing sleep disruption.

EFFECT OF PARKINSON'S DISEASE ON SLEEP

The effect of PD on sleep (Table 13.5) includes sleep initiation and maintenance insomnia; sleep-related respiratory dysrhythmia and sleep fragmentation causing excessive daytime somnolence (EDS); and sleep–wake rhythm alterations (inversion of sleep–wake rhythm), particularly in those patients with dementia. Factors responsible for sleep problems in PD include a patient's inability to turn over at night or on awakening in the middle of the night, leg cramps and jerks, dystonic spasms of the limbs or face, back pain, excessive nocturia, difficulty getting out of bed unaided, and re-emergence of tremor and

Table 13.4
Sleep complaints in Parkinson's disease

Insomnia
Hypersomnia
Parasomnias
Circadian dysrhythmias

Table 13.5
Effect of Parkinson's disease on sleep

Sleep initiation and maintenance insomnia
Sleep-related respiratory dysrhythmia
Sleep fragmentation
Excessive daytime somnolence
Sleep–wake rhythm alterations

---

rigidity in sleep. Sleep disruption is more common in advanced PD than in early PD.

Sleep-related respiratory dysrhythmias (obstructive, central, and mixed apneas) may be more common in PD patients than in age-matched controls. Patients with autonomic dysfunction in PD show increased incidences of sleep-disordered breathing. Sleep apnea–hypopneas in PD may result from an impairment of respiratory muscle function owing to rigidity or an impairment of the central control of breathing. Other factors for sleep-disordered breathing events in PD include laryngeal stridor or spasms associated with off-states or dystonic episodes, diaphragmatic dyskinesias, and upper airway dysfunction.

EFFECT OF SLEEP ON PARKINSON'S DISEASE

Effects of sleep on PD (Table 13.6) include alterations in parkinsonian motor abnormalities (e.g., decreased body movements and positional shifts in sleep and persistence of tremor in lighter stages of sleep or its re-emergence in the transition between sleep and wakefulness and on awakenings), sleep-onset rapid blinking, intrusion of REMs in NREM sleep, REM onset blepharospasms, the presence of PLMS in many PD

Table 13.6
Effect of sleep on Parkinson's disease

Changes in parkinsonian motor abnormalities
Decreased body movements and positional shifts in sleep
Sleep-onset rapid blinking
Intrusion of rapid eye movements (REMs) in nonrapid eye movement sleep
REM-onset blepharospasm
Excessive periodic limb movements in sleep
REM sleep behavior disorder
Sleep benefit: morning improvement of motor features

Table 13.7
Effect of antiparkinsonian drugs on sleep

Respiratory dyskinesias
End-of-the-dose dyskinesia
Peak-dose dyskinesia
Sleep fragmentation

---

patients, REM sleep behavior disorder (RBD), and morning improvement of parkinsonian motor features (sleep benefit) in many patients.

EFFECT OF ANTIPARKINSONIAN MEDICATIONS ON SLEEP
Antiparkinsonian medications may cause respiratory and other dyskinesias, either peak-dose dyskinesias (mainly choreiform), which occur when dopaminergic agents exert their maximum central effects, or end-of-the-dose dyskinesias (mostly dystonic), which occur when the effects of dopaminergic agents are beginning to wane (Table 13.7). These dyskinesias may cause sleep disruption and fragmentation of sleep. Myoclonus, akathisia, and PLMS are other abnormal movements that may be noted after prolonged levodopa therapy. These movements may cause sleep initiation and maintenance problems. Vivid or frightening dreams (and sometimes psychosis) can occur after long-standing dopaminergic treatment, causing sleep maintenance problems and EDS.

ASSOCIATED CONDITIONS CAUSING SLEEP DISRUPTION
   IN PARKINSON'S DISEASE
Secondary sleep disturbances in PD may result from associated depression, dementia, sleep apnea, RLS, PLMS, RBD or other parasomnias (sleepwalking, sleep talking), and the circadian rhythm disturbances seen in some advanced demented PD patients. Some reports suggest a common occurrence of RBD in PD, and, in some cases, RBD precedes parkinsonian symptoms. Details of RBD are described in Chapter 18.

Sleep Disturbances in Other Extrapyramidal Disorders

Significant sleep disruption has been noted in patients with Huntington's disease (HD), progressive supranuclear palsy (PSP), torsion dystonia, and Tourette's syndrome (TS).

   HD is a neurodegenerative disease characterized by dementia, chorea, and a dominant mode of inheritance whose gene has been linked to the short arm of chromosome 4. Onset occurs between 25 and 40 years of age with inexorable and relentless progression. Sleep disturbance has been described in approximately 20% of patients with late-onset HD. Insomnia with impairment of initiation and maintenance of sleep is a common complaint, particularly in moderate to severe cases. As the disease progresses, sleep fragmentation increases, but sleep apnea and EDS are uncommon. Choreiform movements show variable persistences during sleep, most of which are present in NREM stage I or II sleep.

PSP is characterized by dystonia, gait disturbance, and characteristic supranuclear eye movement abnormalities manifested initially by impaired voluntary vertical eye movements, particularly downward gaze with later involvement of eye movements in all directions. Sleep disturbance is present in almost all cases of PSP. Insomnia with difficulty in initiation and maintenance of sleep is a common complaint. Sleep disruption in PSP increases with the severity of motor abnormalities.

Dystonia musculorum deformans, or torsion dystonia, may be hereditary, beginning in childhood, or idiopathic, with onset in early adult life. The disease is characterized by contorting movements and sustained distorting or twisting postures, often intermixed with a variety of more jerky movements. It may be primary or secondary to various causes. In many cases of primary dystonia, a locus at chromosome 9 accounts for inheritance. Sleep disturbances with a progressive deterioration of sleep occur as the disease progresses. Dystonic movements may persist during lighter stages of sleep but are reduced mostly during SWS; they may show partial reactivation during REM sleep. A particular type of dystonia called *dopa-responsive dystonia*, or hereditary progressive dystonia with diurnal fluctuation, often presents before age 10 years and appears to occur mainly in girls. Dystonic posturing of one foot is the most common initial symptom, with a later spread of dystonia to all four limbs. The patient also develops a parkinsonian-type masked face, rigidity, and flexed posture. Significant symptomatic relief from sleep is noted in these patients, who also show dramatic improvement with small doses of levodopa.

Patients with TS present with multiple motor tics that typically are manifested as stereotyped, complex, and often repetitive movements accompanied by vocal tics. Onset occurs during childhood or adolescence and is often familial. Obsessive-compulsive disorder and other behavioral abnormalities may accompany this movement disorder. Tics often persist during sleep, mostly in stages I and II NREM sleep. Sleep disturbances, including parasomnias and respiratory disturbances, occur in 44–80% of patients with TS. Patients may give a history of somnambulism. Other parasomnias, such as night terrors, confusional

Table 13.8
Diagnostic criteria for periodic limb movements in sleep

Repetitive, often stereotyped movements during nonrapid eye movement sleep
Usually noted in the legs, consisting of extension of the great toe, dorsiflexion
  of the ankle, and flexion of the knee and hip; sometimes seen in the arms
Periodic or quasiperiodic at an average interval of 20–40 secs (range, 5–120
  secs) with a duration of 0.5–5.0 secs and as part of at least four consecu-
  tive movements
Occurs at any age but prevalence increases with age
May occur as an isolated condition or may be associated with a large number
  of other medical, neurologic, or sleep disorders and medications
Seen in at least 80% of patients with restless legs syndrome

---

arousals, and nocturnal enuresis, may also occur. Sleep disturbance improves as the patient gets older.

Periodic Limb Movements in Sleep

PLMS is characterized by periodically recurring stereotyped limb movements that occur during NREM sleep; most commonly, patients dorsiflex ankles or flex knees or hips every 20–40 seconds (Table 13.8). Movements generally affect both legs but may predominantly affect one leg or alternate between the two legs. Occasionally, PLMS may be noted in the upper limbs. Most movements occur during NREM stages I and II sleep, but sometimes movements may occur during SWS or REM sleep. In a minority of patients, particularly those with RLS, these movements may occur during the wake state, called *periodic limb movements in wakefulness*. PLMS is generally noted during the first half of the night but sometimes—particularly in PLMS associated with narcolepsy and OSAS—may be evenly distributed throughout the night.

For a diagnosis of PLMS, PSG recordings are essential and criteria have been established. PLMS have periodic or quasiperiodic movements that occur as part of at least four consecutive movements during any sleep stage at intervals of 5–90 seconds (some investigators use intervals of 5–120 seconds), a duration of 0.5–5.0 seconds, and an amplitude of leg electromyographic (EMG) activity that must be at least 25% of the amplitude recorded in a presleep calibration recording. A PLMS index (i.e., the number of PLMS per hour of sleep) of 5 is considered abnormal. The number of PLMS associated with arousals is also counted and is considered to be more significant than those without arousal.

Table 13.9
Conditions associated with periodic limb movements in sleep

Primary sleep disorders
    Obstructive sleep apnea
    Narcolepsy
    Rapid eye movement sleep behavior disorder
Neurologic disorders
    Parkinson's disease
    Peripheral neuropathies
    Spinal cord lesions
    Multiple sclerosis
    Huntington's disease
    Amyotrophic lateral sclerosis
    Lumbosacral radiculopathies
    Isaac's syndrome
    Stiff-man syndrome
    Hyperekplexia
Psychiatric disorders
    Post-traumatic stress disorder
    Akathisia
    Attention-deficit hyperactivity disorder
General medical disorders
    Chronic obstructive pulmonary disease
    Congestive cardiac failure
    Chronic fatigue syndrome
    Fibromyalgia
    Diabetes mellitus
    Leukemia
Medications
    Tricyclic antidepressants
    Serotonin reuptake inhibitors
    Levodopa
Miscellaneous
    Ethanol

PLMS may occur as an isolated condition, called *periodic limb movement disorder* (PLMD), or may be associated with a variety of other medical and neurologic illnesses, medications, or exogenous chemicals as well as a number of primary sleep disorders (Table 13.9). PLMS is noted in at least 80% of cases of RLS syndrome; RLS is noted in approximately 30% of cases of PLMS. PLMS is also common in patients with OSAS and narcolepsy. Medications (tricyclics, serotonin-reuptake blockers, or levodopa) may simply aggravate symptoms rather than trigger movements. In addition, asymptomatic PLMS can occur in normal individuals, particularly in elderly subjects (in whom a prevalence of 30% has been reported). PLMS is most prevalent in middle-aged to elderly patients. Considerable night-to-night variability in severity of PLMS occurs; therefore, its true prevalence is not well known. Furthermore, a dearth of control studies exists. Finally, whether PLMD exists as a primary condition causing sleep maintenance insomnia or excessive sleepiness, or whether it is simply an epiphenomenon and found in a wide variety of conditions causing sleep disturbance remains to be determined.

Restless Legs Syndrome

Despite a lucid description in the 1940s of the entity known as RLS, considerable misconceptions about the condition exist and misdiagnosis occurs. The prevalence of RLS has varied from 1% to 15% and is most likely approximately 4%. Adequate epidemiologic study has not been undertaken. Patients are served mainly by internists, family physicians, neurologists, and sleep specialists. Currently, no single laboratory test to confirm diagnosis exists, and even the clinical criteria for diagnosis were somewhat vague until 1995, when the International RLS Study Group defined a set of clinical criteria for diagnosing RLS.

The fundamental problem of RLS is a complex sensory-motor disorder predominantly involving the legs. Table 13.10 lists the clinical diagnostic criteria for RLS. RLS may be divided into a primary (or idiopathic) form or a secondary form, which is associated with (or in some cases may result from) a variety of causes (Table 13.11).

The International RLS Study Group published four major (minimal) and five ancillary criteria for the diagnosis of RLS (see Table 13.10). Minimal criteria include the following: desire to move the limbs, usually associated with paresthesia or dysesthesia; motor restlessness; worsening of symptoms or exclusive presence at rest (i.e., lying, sitting), with at least partial and temporary relief by activities; and worsening of symptoms in the evening or night. Ancillary criteria, or additional clinical features, include sleep disturbance, involuntary movements, neurologic examination, clinical course, and family history (see Table 13.10).

Sensory manifestations include intensive disagreeable feelings, which are described as creeping, crawling, tingling, burning, painful, aching, cramping, knifelike, or itching sensations. These creeping sensations occur mostly between the knees and ankles, causing an intense urge to move the limbs to relieve these feelings. Occasionally, patients complain of pain.

Table 13.10
Diagnostic criteria for idiopathic restless legs syndrome

Minimal criteria
    Desire to move limbs, usually associated with paresthesia or dysesthesia
    Motor restlessness
    Worsening of symptoms or exclusive presence at rest (i.e., sitting or lying
        down) with at least partial and temporary relief by motor activity
    Worsening of symptoms in the evening or night, suggesting a circadian
        variability
Ancillary criteria
    Involuntary movements
        Periodic limb movements in sleep (may also occur while at rest in
            wakefulness)
        Myoclonic and dystonic leg movements in relaxed wakefulness, which
            may be periodic or aperiodic
    Sleep disturbance, especially difficulty in initiating sleep
    Normal neurologic examination (in secondary restless legs syndrome, may
        be abnormal depending on potential causes or associations)
    Autosomal dominant inheritance
    The course is typically chronic and progressive, with occasional remission
        and frequent aggravation during pregnancy; onset at any age; most
        severe in middle-aged and elderly individuals

Motor restlessness is observed mostly in the legs but occasionally also in the arms. This condition generally involves tossing and turning in bed, floor pacing, leg stretching, leg flexion, foot rubbing, and, occasionally, marching in place and body rocking. Involuntary movements noted during relaxed wakefulness include myoclonic jerks (i.e., brief muscle jerks) and dystonic movements, which are more sustained and prolonged in duration than myoclonic jerks. The most important involuntary movements are PLMS (see Table 13.9). PLMS are noted in at least 80% of patients with RLS. PLMS may sometimes be observed also during wakefulness. PLMS are mostly dystonic and rarely myoclonic, based on the EMG criteria of duration of muscle bursts. Most commonly, the symptoms occur during the evening or early part of the night. In severe cases, symptoms may occur even in relaxed conditions during the day.

Sleep disturbances in RLS are generally a problem of initiation, but difficulty maintaining sleep because of associated PLMS also occurs in 80% of the cases.

Neurologic examination of the primary or idiopathic form is generally normal, as most of the time movements (at least in the early stage)

Table 13.11
Causes of secondary restless legs syndrome

Neurologic disorders
    Polyneuropathies
    Lumbosacral radiculopathies
    Amyotrophic lateral sclerosis
    Myelopathies
    Multiple sclerosis
    Parkinson's disease
    Poliomyelitis
    Isaac's syndrome
    Hyperekplexia (startle disease)
Medical disorders
    Anemia (iron and folate deficiency)
    Diabetes mellitus
    Amyloidosis
    Uremia
    Gastrectomy
    Cancer
    Chronic obstructive pulmonary disease
    Peripheral vascular (arterial or venous) disorder
    Rheumatoid arthritis
    Hypothyroidism
Drugs and chemicals
    Caffeine
    Neuroleptics
    Withdrawal from sedatives or narcotics
    Lithium
    Calcium channel antagonists (e.g., nifedipine)

---

are noted in the evening while patients are resting in bed. In severe cases, however, movements may be noted in the daytime while subjects are sitting or lying down; voluntary and involuntary movements may be seen during neurologic examination. In the secondary forms of RLS, clinical signs of an associated abnormality (see Table 13.11) may be present.

Onset of disease occurs at any age but most severe cases are noted in middle-aged and elderly subjects. A few cases have been described in children, and a reported association between childhood RLS and attention-deficit hyperactivity disorder exists. The course is generally chronic and progressive, but sometimes remissions occur. The condition may be exacerbated during pregnancy, by caffeine or iron deficiency. The most important associations of RLS with pathologic

Table 13.12
Conditions mimicking restless legs syndrome

Neuroleptic-induced akathisia
Syndrome of painful legs and moving toes
Muscular pain-fasciculation syndrome
Myokymia
Causalgia-dystonia syndrome
Painful nocturnal leg cramps
Myoclonus (essential myoclonus)
Hypnic jerks ("sleep starts")
Anxiety or depression
Growing pains

---

conditions are iron deficiency (with or without frank anemia), uremia, polyneuropathy (particularly that associated with diabetes mellitus), and rheumatoid arthritis. Iron deficiency is an important provocative factor for RLS; treating iron deficiency (best measured by serum ferritin level) can improve symptoms or patient response to other RLS medications. Family history may be present in 30–50% of patients, suggesting a dominant mode of inheritance exists.

The differential diagnosis of RLS may be considered under two categories: secondary RLS and the entities that mimic RLS. In secondary or symptomatic RLS (see Table 13.11), several conditions exist that may be associated with RLS or that may cause symptomatic RLS. The entities that may mimic RLS are listed in Table 13.12. An important and often difficult condition to differentiate from RLS is akathisia (Table 13.13).

The physiologic mechanism or locus responsible for RLS–PLMS pathology is unknown. Based on pharmacologic response, dopaminergic theory has received the most support. Other theories, such as vascular, peripheral neuropathy, and deficiency or toxic hypotheses, have not been satisfactorily proven. The most likely hypothesis is that a functional alteration exists in the brain stem region, but its exact location is undetermined. A circadian factor modulating RLS severity independent of activity state has been postulated, based on findings that RLS symptoms are maximum during the falling phase of a body temperature curve.

Approach to a Patient with Movement Disorders during Sleep

An approach to treating a patient complaining of excessive or abnormal movements (which can be either physiologic or pathologic) dur-

Table 13.13
Salient features of akathisia that differentiate from restless legs syndrome

---

Inner restlessness, fidgetiness with jittery feelings, or generalized restlessness.

Common side effect of neuroleptics.

Can be acute, chronic, or tardive.

Characteristic motor restlessness consists of swaying or rocking movements of the body, marching in place, crossing and uncrossing of legs, shifting body positions in chair, inability to sit still, rhythmic or nonrhythmic, synchronous or asynchronous, symmetric or asymmetric limb movements. Movements resemble chorea rather than voluntary movements of restless legs syndrome.

Motor restlessness is present mostly during the day but may be worse when sitting or standing in one place for a long time.

Polysomnographic study shows no distinctive features or rarely may show evidence of mild sleep disturbance and periodic leg movements in sleep.

No relevant family history.

Neurologic examination reveals evidence of akathisia and (sometimes) drug-induced extrapyramidal manifestations.

Involuntary movements, such as myoclonic jerks, are uncommon and are not a prominent feature.

Best treated with anticholinergics or β-adrenergic antagonists.

---

ing or at the onset of sleep at night should begin with a careful history from patients, parents, bed partners, or caregivers. Particular attention should be paid to the description of the motor events and the occurrence at onset (e.g., restless legs syndrome occurring before sleep and hypnic jerks occurring at sleep onset) during the first third of the night (e.g., NREM motor parasomnias and nocturnal seizures), the last third of the night (e.g., RBD or nightmares), or throughout the night (e.g., sleep apnea with repeated awakenings and body movements, bruxism, neonatal sleep myoclonus, excessive fragmentary myoclonus, and diurnal involuntary movements reappearing during sleep). A thorough physical examination should direct attention to any underlying structural causes of abnormal movements or uncover the presence of characteristics typical of diurnal movement disorders.

Laboratory assessment for patients with parasomnias or nocturnal seizures, important conditions that should be considered in the differential diagnosis of abnormal movements during sleep at night, has been discussed in Chapters 14 and 18.

In RLS patients, EMG and nerve conduction studies are important to exclude polyneuropathies, lumbosacral radiculopathies, or other lower motor neuron disorders that may either be associated with RLS or cause symptoms resembling idiopathic RLS. Other important laboratory tests in RLS include those necessary to obtain appropriate tests to exclude diabetes mellitus, uremia, anemia, and other associated conditions. Obtaining levels of serum iron (including serum ferritin), serum folate levels, fasting blood glucose, blood urea, and creatinine is particularly important.

Management of Patients with Movement Disorders and Sleep Disturbance

Determining a cause for sleep disturbance so that the primary condition can be adequately treated is important. Treatment of secondary sleep disturbances is unlikely to be successful unless the primary cause is properly diagnosed and treated. Treatment of an underlying cause may improve sleep disturbance. If satisfactory treatment is not available for the primary condition or does not resolve the problem, however, treatment should be directed to the specific sleep disturbance. Certain general principles, including following sleep hygiene measures, should apply to treatment of any sleep disorders. Management of parasomnias and nocturnal seizures have been discussed in Chapters 14 and 18. In this section, management of sleep disturbances in patients with PD and RLS–PLMS is reviewed. Sleep-related breathing disorders in PD and parkinsonism have been described in Chapter 14.

Management of Sleep Disturbance in Patients with Parkinson's Disease

Treatment of PD has not been found to improve sleep consistently. Some patients report parallel sleep and motor abnormality benefits, whereas others note persistent abnormalities in sleep. Adjustment in timing and choice of medications may be helpful in those patients who experience a reactivation of parkinsonian motor symptoms during sleep. A bedtime dose of a dopaminergic agent, especially in advanced cases with severe motor abnormalities during sleep, may result in improved motility and better sleep. Longer-acting preparations of levodopa (Sinemet CR) or dopamine agonists (e.g., bromocriptine or pergolide) with sustained actions may benefit sleep in some patients. A small dose of carbidopa–levodopa, with a second dose administered later at night if the patient awakens, may sometimes help patients who experience insomnia. Higher doses, however, may disrupt sleep by causing repeated awakenings or arousals, vivid dreams, or hallucinations. PD patients with RLS–PLMS may benefit from evening and late-night doses of levodopa. Sometimes, such patients require small doses of clonazepam, pergolide, or codeine to control PLMS associated with arousal and sleep disturbance.

Patients with nocturnal hallucinations and nightmares, including nocturnal vocalizations and RBD, may benefit from a small dose of clonazepam (0.5–1.0 mg) at bedtime. Nocturnal hallucinations and psychosis in PD patients have been treated successfully with clozapine or olanzapine. During clozapine treatment, usual precautions of monitoring blood count and testing liver function should be taken.

Sleep-disordered breathing is not improved by levodopa treatment, and in severe cases with moderate to marked oxygen desaturation, a trial of continuous positive airway pressure (CPAP) titration may be beneficial.

Management of Restless Legs Syndrome–Periodic Limb Movements in Sleep

Four major groups of drugs have been used to treat RLS–PLMS (Table 13.14): dopaminergic agents, benzodiazepines, gabapentin, and opiates.

Table 13.14
Drug treatment of restless legs syndrome

Major drugs
  Dopaminergic agents
    Carbidopa–levodopa
    Pergolide
    Bromocriptine
    Pramipexole
    Ropinirole
  Benzodiazepines
    Clonazepam
    Temazepam
  Gabapentin
  Opiates
    Codeine
    Propoxyphene
    Oxycodone
    Methadone
Minor drugs
  Tramadol
  Baclofen
  Carbamazepine
  Clonidine
  Propranolol

The typical dose for carbidopa–levodopa (Sinemet CR) is 25/100 to 100/400 mg, taken in divided doses before bedtime and during the night. Pergolide can be started at 0.05 mg and gradually increased to 0.20–0.50 mg, taken in divided doses. One dose is taken an hour before bedtime; depending on the severity, another dose may be needed earlier in the evening or during the middle of the night on awakening. Another dopamine agonist, bromocriptine, may be administered, beginning with 2.5 mg and gradually increasing to a maximum of 15 mg per day. Some- times a long-acting drug (e.g., Sinemet CR) may be combined with short- acting carbidopa–levodopa (Sinemet) for maximum benefit. The problem with the use of dopaminergic medications include abdominal pain, nau- sea, vomiting, headache, recurrence of RLS symptoms, and poor sleep quality during the last part of the night. Nasal stuffiness, hypotension, and nightmares have been reported, particularly after pergolide use. Two other major problems have been noted after dopaminergic treatment: rebound, which is characterized by the tendency of symptoms to recur late in the night, leading to poor sleep quality near the morning; and augmentation, which causes symptoms to develop early in the day (e.g., in the late afternoon instead of mid-evening) and to be more severe than before treatment. Two new dopamine agonists, pramipexole and ropini- role, have been approved by the U.S. Food and Drug Administration for treatment of PD. Initial reports suggest that these newly approved dopamine agonists are useful in RLS. Pramipexole may be started with 0.125 mg at bedtime and gradually increased to a maximum of 1 mg. Doses have not been established yet for ropinirole.

Clonazepam (0.5–2.0 mg at bedtime) or temazepam (15–30 mg at bedtime) may be useful in treating RLS–PLMS, particularly in those patients with primary complaints of sleep dysfunction. The lowest doses of these medications should be initially administered, then grad- ually increased to obtain maximum benefits with minimal side effects. These agents may produce daytime sleepiness or confusional episodes, particularly in elderly patients.

Gabapentin is an anticonvulsant that has been found to be benefi- cial in mild-to-moderate cases of RLS–PLMS, particularly in patients complaining of pain associated with RLS. Divided doses of 300–1,800 mg per day may be helpful but can produce somnolence, dizziness, ataxia, or fatigue in more than 10% of patients. Opiates are effective for treating RLS–PLMS but are less desirable alternatives because of their addictive potential and proclivity to produce constipation. Codeine, propoxyphene, oxycodone, and methadone have all been used to treat RLS–PLMS. Tramadol, a non-narcotic agent with activity at the opiate mu receptor, also has been used with some success in patients with RLS–PLMS.

In mild-to-moderate cases, patients may start with gabapentin. In moderate-to-severe cases, carbidopa–levodopa is the first treatment of choice; however, some physicians elect to use clonazepam. In refractory cases, patients may have to use a combination of two to three drugs.

Overall, the principle for treating RLS–PLMS is to begin with the lowest possible dose and then increase it every 5–6 days until a maximum therapeutic benefit is achieved or side effects are noted. Doses can be divided and given 1–2 hours before bedtime, at bedtime, and in the middle of the night. If necessary, and in some severe cases, a daytime dose may be needed.

Other minor drugs (see Table 13.14) that have been helpful occasionally in patients with RLS–PLMS include baclofen (10–60 mg daily), carbamazepine (200–600 mg daily), clonidine, an adrenergic agent (0.1–0.9 mg daily), and propranolol (80–120 mg daily).

In secondary RLS, the primary condition should be treated and deficiency states (including iron deficiency) should be corrected. Patients should also follow general sleep hygiene measures. Finally, patients should avoid certain medications and agents that may aggravate RLS, including neuroleptics, tricyclics, selective serotonin reuptake inhibitors, certain antiemetic medications, calcium channel blockers, caffeine, alcohol, and smoking.

14

Sleep and Neurologic Disorders

Coexistence of neurologic disorders and sleep dysfunction is common. An adverse interaction between neurologic illness and sleep dysfunction exists. Neurologic disorders may cause a variety of sleep disturbances, and sleep disorders may have profound deleterious effects on natural courses of neurologic illnesses. Sleep dysfunction may result from central or peripheral somatic or autonomic neurologic disorders. Neurologic diseases may cause insomnia or excessive daytime somnolence (EDS) as well as parasomnias and circadian rhythm disorders.

Neurologic causes of insomnia have been described in Chapter 11. Insomnia results from direct and indirect pathogenetic mechanisms. The delicate balance between waking and sleeping brain may be altered, causing sleeplessness as a result of lesions of hypnogenic neurons in the hypothalamic–preoptic nuclei and the lower brain stem in the region of the nucleus tractus solitarius. Sleep can also be disturbed in neurologic conditions that cause pain, confusional episodes, changes in the sensorimotor system, or movement disorders. Sleep-related hypoventilation and sleep fragmentation may cause insomnia in some neuromuscular diseases, but most patients who experience it have EDS. Drugs used to treat neurologic illness (e.g., anticonvulsants, dopaminergic agents, anticholinergics) may cause insomnia.

Neurologic disorders may also cause hypersomnia (Table 14.1). Daytime sleepiness can result from tumors and vascular lesions affecting the ascending reticular activating arousal system and its projections to the posterior hypothalamus and thalamus. Such lesions often cause coma rather than sleepiness, however. Other causes of excessive sleepiness may include astrocytomas, suprasellar cysts, metastatic tumors, lymphomas, and hamartomas affecting the posterior hypothalamus, and pineal tumors and astrocytomas of the upper brain stem. Third ventricular tumors may cause prolonged hypersomnia. Symptomatic narcolepsy has occasionally resulted from craniopharyngioma and other tumors of the hypothalamic and pituitary regions, rostral brain

Table 14.1
Neurologic causes of hypersomnia

Brain tumor
Stroke
Encephalitis
Encephalopathies, including Wernicke's encephalopathy
Post-traumatic hypersomnolence
Multiple sclerosis
Neurodegenerative disorders (e.g., Alzheimer's disease, multiple system
   atrophy, Parkinson's disease)
Neuromuscular disorders (e.g., myotonic dystrophy)
Cerebral trypanosomiasis ("African sleeping sickness")
Epilepsy

---

stem gliomas, multiple sclerosis, arteriovenous malformations of the diencephalon, and cerebral sarcoidosis involving the hypothalamus. Finally, encephalitis and encephalopathies, neurodegenerative diseases, and neuromuscular disorders may cause EDS.

NEURODEGENERATIVE DISORDERS

Degenerative diseases of the nervous system generally affect one or more systems symmetrically, running inexorably progressive courses for which no causal agent can be identified by available diagnostic techniques. These disorders include conditions that cause progressive dementia with or without disorders of posture or other associated neurologic deficits, those characterized by progressive cerebellar or spinocerebellar ataxias with or without extrapyramidal or lower motor neuron dysfunction, those causing progressive autonomic failure with or without multiple somatic neurologic deficits, and those that cause degeneration of motor neurons. Parkinson's disease and other extrapyramidal disorders have been described in Chapter 13.

Alzheimer's Disease

Alzheimer's disease (AD) is the most common cerebral degenerative disorder causing dementia. Reports of sleep disturbance in AD are contradictory. Sleep dysfunction in AD may be related to severity of dementia, associated periodic limb movements in sleep (PLMS), or sleep-related respiratory dysrhythmias. Insomnia, inversion of sleep rhythm, and in some cases, EDS, are the presenting complaints. Sleep dysfunction in AD should be differentiated from that which occurs in depression and is common in elderly subjects. A reduction in amount of REM sleep and reduced REM density (as noted in many cases of AD) are quite different from the reduced REM latency and increased REM density that are seen often in depressed patients. Sleep-related respiratory dysrhythmia has been estimated to be present in 33–53% of AD patients. Whether an increased prevalence of sleep apnea exists and whether sleep apnea increases with severity of illness or rapid disease progression remains to be determined. "Sundowning" is a major problem in many AD patients, causing episodes of nocturnal confusion that are often accompanied by a partial or complete inversion of sleep rhythms with increased wakefulness at night and sleepiness in the daytime. Mechanisms of sleep disturbances in AD include the degeneration of neurons of the suprachiasmatic nuclei, cholinergic neurons in the nucleus basalis of Meynert, pedunculopontine tegmental and laterodorsal tegmental nuclei, and brain stem noradrenergic neurons. Associated depression, PLMS, general medical disorders, medication effects, and environmental factors all play significant roles in the pathogenesis of sleep disturbance in AD.

Predominantly Cerebellar or Cerebellar Plus Syndrome

Sleep disturbance may occur in many patients with olivopontocerebellar atrophy (OCPA) and other types of spinocerebellar ataxias (SCAs). Although several genes with expanded CAG repeats responsible for autosomal dominant cerebellar ataxia in SCAs have been described, approximately 40% of dominant ataxias have not been identified at a genotypic level. Cases of recessive or sporadic OPCA are classified under multiple system atrophy (MSA). Central, upper airway obstructive, or mixed sleep apneas are described in many patients with OPCA, but apneas are less frequent and less intense in this condition than in MSA. Typical features of rapid eye movement sleep behavior disorder (RBD) are described in patients with OPCA. Sleep initiation and maintenance problems are other complaints of patients with SCAs (particularly those with SCA3). Patients with SCA3 may also have a high prevalence of restless legs syndrome.

Multiple System Atrophy

In a consensus conference, the term *MSA* was suggested to replace *Shy-Drager syndrome*. MSA is defined as sporadic adult-onset multisystem neurodegenerative disease that initially presents with progressive autonomic failure, followed by progressive somatic neurologic manifestations affecting multiple systems—in particular, the cerebellar and extrapyramidal pathways (Table 14.2). The term *striatonigral degeneration* is used to describe a condition in which the predominant feature is parkinsonism, whereas *OPCA* is used when cerebellar features are the predominant manifestations. The term *Shy-Drager syndrome* is still used to describe a condition in which autonomic failure is the predominant feature. Some patients complain of insomnia and occasionally manifest RBD, but the most common sleep dysfunction in MSA results from sleep-related respiratory dysrhythmia associated with repeated arousals and hypoxemia. A variety of sleep-related respiratory disturbances may occur, including obstructive, central, and mixed apneas and hypopneas; dysrhythmic breathing; Cheyne-Stokes breathing; and nocturnal inspiratory stridor. Sudden nocturnal death in patients with MSA, presumably owing to cardiorespiratory arrest, is reported in some cases. Polysomnographic (PSG) study of MSA may show a reduction in total sleep time, decreased sleep efficiency, increased number of awakenings during sleep, reductions of slow wave sleep (SWS) or rapid eye movement (REM) sleep, absence of muscle atonia in REM sleep in those with RBD, and a variety of respiratory dysrhythmias. Sleep disruption in MSA may result from direct and indirect pathogenetic mechanisms, which may include the following: degeneration of sleep–wake generating neurons in the brain stem and hypothalamus, degeneration of respiratory neurons or direct involvement of projections from the hypothalamus and central nucleus of amygdala to the respiratory neurons in the nucleus tractus solitarius and nucleus ambiguus, interference with vagal inputs from peripheral respiratory receptors to central respiratory neurons, sympathetic denervation of nasal mucosa, and alteration of the neurochemical environment.

Degenerative Diseases of Motor Neurons

Motor neuron disease, also known as *amyotrophic lateral sclerosis* (ALS), may cause daytime hypersomnolence as a result of repeated sleep-related apneas, hypopneas, hypoxemia, hypercapnia, and sleep fragmentation. Some patients complain of insomnia. Sleep-related breathing dysrhythmias in ALS may result from weakness of the upper airway, diaphragmatic, and intercostal muscles due to involvement of the bulbar, phrenic, and intercostal motor nuclei. Additionally, degeneration of central respiratory neurons may occur, causing central and obstructive sleep apneas in ALS.

Table 14.2
Salient clinical features of multiple system atrophy

Autonomic features
  Cardiovascular
    Orthostatic hypotension
    Postprandial hypotension
    Postural syncope
    Postural dizziness, faint feelings, or blurring of vision
    Orthostatic intolerance
  Genitourinary
    Urinary bladder dysfunction (incontinence, hesitancy, frequency, nocturia)
    Impotence in men
  Sudomotor
    Hypohidrosis or anhidrosis
  Gastrointestinal
    Gastroparesis
    Intermittent diarrhea or constipation (intestinal or colonic dysmotility)
    Abnormal swallowing (esophageal dysmotility)
  Ocular
    Horner's syndrome
    Unequal pupils
Nonautonomic manifestations
  Parkinsonism
    Rigidity
    Bradykinesia or akinesia
    Postural instability
  Cerebellar dysfunction
    Ataxic gait
    Scanning speech
    Dysmetria
    Dysdiadochokinesia
    Intention tremor
  Upper motor neuron signs
    Extensor plantar responses
    Hyperreflexia
    Spasticity
  Lower motor neuron signs
    Muscle wasting
    Fasciculations
  Respiratory
    Sleep apnea–hypopnea
    Other respiratory dysrhythmias
  Normal mentation
  Normal sensation

STROKE AND SLEEP DISTURBANCES

Sleep disruption and sleep complaints are described in patients with cerebral hemispheric, paramedian thalamic, and brain stem infarction. In some patients, insomnia may result from associated depression, spasticity, and immobility with repeated awakenings. Based on case control, epidemiologic and laboratory studies, increasing evidence that sleep apnea, snoring, and stroke are intimately related exists; sleep apnea may predispose patients to stroke, and stroke may predispose patients to sleep apnea. An increased frequency of sleep apnea is noted in patients with infratentorial and supratentorial strokes. Several confounding variables exist, however, that are common risk factors for snoring, sleep apnea, and stroke (e.g., hypertension, cardiac disease, age, body mass index, smoking, and alcohol intake). These variables should be considered when attempting to establish a relationship between snoring, sleep apnea, and stroke. It is important to make a diagnosis of sleep apnea in stroke patients because it may adversely affect their short- and long-term outcomes. Effective treatment for sleep apnea that can decrease risk of future stroke exists.

Brain stem infarction may cause the syndrome known as *Ondine's curse*, or primary failure of automatic respiration. Metabolic control, the only respiratory control used during sleep, is impaired in these patients, but voluntary breathing control is intact. Therefore, patients become apneic during sleep. This syndrome is usually caused by bilateral lesions caudal to the fifth cranial nerve in the pons down to the upper cervical spinal cord in the ventrolateral region. Occasional patients with unilateral brain stem infarctions experience a loss of automatic respiratory control during sleep.

SLEEP AND EPILEPSY

A reciprocal relationship exists between sleep and epilepsy (i.e., sleep affects epilepsy, and epilepsy, in turn, affects sleep). Most of the time, seizures are triggered during nonrapid eye movement (NREM) stages I and II sleep; however, they are occasionally triggered during NREM stages III and IV sleep. In epilepsy, NREM sleep acts as a convulsant causing excessive synchronization and activation of seizures in an already hyperexcitable cortex. In contrast, during REM sleep, an attenuation of epileptiform discharges and limitation of propagation of generalized epileptiform discharges to a focal area occurs. Sleep deprivation is another important seizure-triggering factor. Sleep deprivation increases epileptiform discharges, mostly during the transition period between waking and light sleep. Sleep deprivation causes sleepiness, one seizure-activating factor, but it probably also increases cortical excitability, which triggers seizures.

Seizures may occur predominantly during sleep (nocturnal seizure), in the daytime (diurnal seizures), or during sleep at night and in the daytime (diffuse epilepsy). Approximately 10% of epileptic patients experience nocturnal seizures. Because inconsistencies and contradictions exist in biorhythmic classification of seizures, however, modern epileptologists use the International Classification of Epilepsy, which divides seizures into three categories: (1) primarily generalized, (2) partial seizures, with or without secondary generalization, and (3) unclassified epileptic seizures.

Effect of Sleep on Epilepsy

Certain types of seizures are characteristically observed during sleep, including tonic seizures, benign focal epilepsy of childhood with rolandic spikes, juvenile myoclonic epilepsy, electrical status epilepticus during sleep, and some varieties of frontal lobe seizures (particularly nocturnal paroxysmal dystonia [NPD]). Some patients with generalized tonic-clonic and partial complex seizures also have predominantly nocturnal seizures. It is important to differentiate nocturnal seizures from motor and behavioral parasomnias or other movement disorders that persist during sleep or reactivate during stage transition or awakenings in the middle of the night.

Tonic Seizures

Tonic seizures are typically activated by sleep, occur much more frequently during NREM sleep than during wakefulness, and are never seen during REM sleep. Typical electroencephalogram (EEG) shows interictal abnormalities during sleep occurring as slow spikes and waves intermixed with trains of fast spikes.

Benign Focal Epilepsy of Childhood

Benign focal epilepsy of childhood (rolandic seizure) is characterized by focal clonic facial twitching that is often preceded by perioral numbness, seen most frequently during drowsiness and sleep. Many patients may have secondary generalized tonic-clonic seizures. Characteristic EEG findings consist of centrotemporal or rolandic spikes or sharp

Table 14.3
Nocturnal paroxysmal dystonia

Onset: infancy to fifth decade of life
Usually sporadic; rarely familial
Sudden onset from nonrapid eye movement sleep
Two clinical types
    Common type is short-lasting (15 secs to <2 mins)
    Rare type is longer lasting (2 mins to <1 hr)
Semiology: ballismic, choreoathetotic, or dystonic movements
Often occurs in clusters
Electroencephalograms: generally normal
Short duration attacks are most likely a type of frontal lobe seizure
Treatment: carbamazepine effective in patients with short-lasting attacks

---

waves. Seizures generally stop by age 15–20 years without any neurologic deficits.

Juvenile Myoclonic Epilepsy

Juvenile myoclonic epilepsy occurs between the ages of 13 and 19 years, manifested by massive bilaterally synchronous myoclonic jerks. These seizures increase shortly after patients awaken in the morning or, occasionally, in the middle of the night. A typical EEG shows synchronous and symmetric multiple spikes and spike and wave discharges.

Electrical Status Epilepticus during Sleep

Electrical status epilepticus during sleep is a childhood disease characterized by generalized continuous slow spike and wave discharges in EEG, seen during at least 85% of NREM sleep and suppressed during REM sleep.

Nocturnal Paroxysmal Dystonia

NPD is characterized by a variety of dystonic, ballismic, and choreoathetotic motor phenomena occurring during NREM sleep (Table 14.3). NPD, particularly the short-duration attack that occurs and lasts less than a minute, is recognized increasingly as a form of frontal lobe seizure evoked specifically during sleep at night (Table 14.4).

Table 14.4
Frontal lobe seizure

Age of onset: infancy to middle age
Sporadic, occasionally familial (dominant)
Both diurnal and nocturnal spells, sometimes exclusively nocturnal
Sudden onset in nonrapid eye movement sleep with sudden termination
Duration: mostly less than 1 min, sometimes 1–2 mins with short postictal
   confusion
Often occurs in clusters
Semiology: tonic, clonic, bipedal, bimanual, and bicycling movements; motor
   and sexual automatisms; contralateral dystonic posturing or arm abduc-
   tion with or without eye deviation
Ictal electroencephalogram may be normal; interictal electroencephalogram
   may show spikes; sometimes depth recording is needed

Nonepileptic seizures, or pseudoseizures, are uncommon during sleep
at night, but sometimes can occur (Table 14.5) and be mistaken for true
nocturnal seizures. It is important to differentiate pseudoseizures from
true seizures because they must be managed differently.

Two other entities—paroxysmal arousals and awakenings and
episodic nocturnal wanderings—share common features of abnormal
paroxysmal motor activities during sleep with NPD, and they all
respond favorably to carbamazepine.

Table 14.5
Nonepileptic seizure (pseudoseizure)

Can be mistaken for true nocturnal seizure
Gradual onset with gradual termination
No postictal confusion
Out-of-phase clonic movements
Forward pelvic thrust
Repetitive stereotyped bizarre movements
To-and-fro head movements without eye deviation
Duration: longer than several minutes
Ictal and interictal electroencephalogram: normal
May also have true seizures (15–20% in some monitoring units)

Autosomal Dominant Nocturnal Frontal Lobe Epilepsy

Autosomal dominant nocturnal frontal lobe epilepsy is a disorder that starts in childhood and persists throughout adult life, characterized by brief motor seizures occurring in clusters during sleep. Neurologic examination and neuroimaging studies are normal. Videotelemetry during attacks confirms their epileptic nature, and their response to carbamazepine is excellent.

Effect of Epilepsy on Sleep

The effects of epilepsy on sleep architecture remain somewhat controversial, although the usefulness of sleep in the diagnosis of epilepsy is well established. Most studies have been conducted in patients who have been taking anticonvulsants, which adds to the results of the confounding factors of anticonvulsant effects on sleep architecture. A general consensus about the effects of epilepsy on sleep and sleep architecture has been reached, however. PSG findings can be summarized as follows: sleep-onset latency increases; an increase in waking after sleep onset occurs; REM sleep is reduced; the instability of sleep states, such as unclassifiable epochs, is increased; an increase in NREM stages I and II occurs; NREM sleep stages III and IV decrease; and a reduction in the density of sleep spindles occurs.

NEUROMUSCULAR DISORDERS

Sleep disorders have been described in many patients with neuromuscular disorders, including myotonic dystrophy and other primary muscle diseases, motor neuron disease or ALS, and neuromuscular junctional disorders and polyneuropathies. The most common sleep complaints among patients are EDS resulting from repeated arousals and sleep fragmentation associated with sleep apnea–hypopnea and hypoventilation. Sleep disturbance in these conditions generally results from involvement of respiratory muscles or phrenic and intercostal nerves, or from neuromuscular junctions of respiratory and oropharyngeal muscles. Additionally, some patients (particularly those with painful neuropathies, muscle pain, muscle cramps, and immobility due to muscle weakness), may complain of insomnia.

Many reports of central, mixed, and upper airway obstructive sleep apneas, alveolar hypoventilation, daytime fatigue, and EDS occur in patients with myotonic dystrophy. In the advanced stage of myotonic dystrophy, nocturnal oxygen desaturation accompanies alveolar hypoventilation and apneas, becoming worse during REM sleep. Sometimes EDS in myotonic dystrophy occurs in the absence of sleep apnea. Sleep disturbance has also been reported in patients with proximal myotonic myopathy, a condition differentiated from classic myotonic dystrophy by the absence of chromosome 19 CTG trinucleotide repeat. The mechanism of sleep apnea in myotonic dystrophy includes both respiratory muscle dysfunction and affection of respiratory and hypnogenic neurons in the brain stem as parts of the generalized membrane disorder.

Respiratory disturbance is generally noted in advanced stages of primary muscle disorders. Sleep complaints and sleep-related respiratory dysrhythmias are commonly seen in patients with Duchenne's and limb-girdle muscular dystrophies and myopathies associated with acid maltase deficiency, and they may also occur in other congenital or acquired myopathies, mitochondrial encephalopathy, and polymyositis.

In polyneuropathies, involvement of the nerves supplying the diaphragm, intercostal, and auxiliary muscles of respiration may cause respiratory dysrhythmias that become worse during sleep, causing sleep fragmentation and daytime hypersomnolence. Patients with painful polyneuropathies may experience insomnia.

Patients with myasthenia gravis may experience central, obstructive, and mixed apneas and hypopneas accompanied by oxygen desaturation. Sleep-related hypoventilation and sleep apnea in neuromuscular junctional disorders may be severe enough to require assisted ventilation.

SLEEP DISTURBANCE IN POLIOMYELITIS AND POSTPOLIO SYNDROME

Sleep-related breathing dysrhythmias causing sleep disturbances are well known in patients during the acute and convalescent stage of poliomyelitis. Sleep disorders in postpolio syndrome, however, are less well known. Patients with postpolio syndrome present with increasing weakness or wasting of previously affected muscles and additional involvement of previously unaffected regions of the body. Patients also experience fatigue, aches and pains, and may experience sleep-related hypoventilation or apnea causing EDS or fatigue.

SPINAL CORD DISEASES

Sleep dysfunction related to respiratory dysrhythmia occurs in some patients with high cervical spinal cord lesions, including patients who have undergone spinal surgery. The most common symptom is hypersomnia secondary to sleep apnea. Occasionally, patients may complain of insomnia as a result of immobility, spasticity associated with flexor spasms, neck pain, and central pain syndromes.

MULTIPLE SCLEROSIS

Many patients with multiple sclerosis present with sleep disturbances resulting from sleep-related breathing dysfunctions, immobility, leg muscle spasms, pain, nocturia, and medications. Sleep complaints include insomnia and EDS.

SLEEP AND HEADACHE SYNDROMES

Headache and sleep complaints are common. Under the heading "Sleep-Related Headaches," the International Classification of Sleep Disorders lists cluster headaches, chronic paroxysmal hemicrania, and migraines. Migraines may occur during sleep or wakefulness. Cluster headaches, severe unilateral headaches that occur more frequently during sleep at night than in daytime, are noted predominantly in men. A cluster headache is characterized by severe excruciating pain occurring around one eye and on the temple of the same side, accompanied by increased lacrimation, conjunctival injection, nasal stuffiness, rhinorrhea, and increased sweating of the forehead on the same side as the headache. Attacks usually last a few hours. PSG recording in patients with migraines and cluster headaches shows a clear relationship exists between REM sleep and attacks of headache, although sometimes migraine headaches with arousal may occur out of both SWS and REM sleep. Cluster headaches are thought to be REM-related but may sometimes be triggered by NREM sleep. Chronic paroxysmal hemicrania, probably a variant of cluster headache, is most commonly associated with REM sleep.

Sleep apnea, particularly REM-related sleep apnea, may trigger cluster headaches. An increased prevalence of sleep apnea occurs in cluster headaches, and patients also may experience sleep maintenance insomnia because of awakening with cluster headaches.

Hypnic headache syndrome is a rare benign-type headache described in patients older than age 60 years. These patients are awakened from sleep at a constant time each night. Hypnic headache syndrome is differentiated from chronic cluster headache by generalized distribution, age of onset, and lack of autonomic manifestations. Patients respond to lithium treatment.

Exploding headache syndrome is an unusual phenomenon occurring during the wake-to-sleep transition that abruptly arouses patients with the sound of an explosion inside the head. It is a benign condition that may represent a form of hypnic jerk.

TRAUMATIC BRAIN INJURIES

Patients with traumatic brain injuries may present with insomnia, hypersomnia, or circadian rhythm dysfunctions. Some patients with postconcussion syndrome may develop sleep–wake abnormalities. Sleep maintenance insomnia, with its increased number of awakenings and decreased total sleep time, sometimes occurs after closed head injury. Other sleep disturbances are post-traumatic hypersomnolence and sleep apnea. Occasionally, post-traumatic delayed sleep phase syndrome is reported.

KLEINE-LEVIN SYNDROME

Periodic hypersomnolence associated with bulimia, as described by Kleine and Levin, affects mostly adolescent boys but is also described in girls. During sleep "attacks," a patient sleeps 16–18 hours per day or more; on awakening, he or she eats voraciously. Other abnormal behavior or disturbances that occur during and after these episodes include hypersexuality, polydipsia, memory impairment, confusion, and hallucination. PSG study shows normal sleep cycling and Multiple Sleep Latency Test (MSLT) shows pathologic sleepiness without sleep onset REM. The cause of the condition is undetermined, although a limbic-hypothalamic dysfunction is suspected, but has not been proven, as a factor. Lithium treatment is effective in many patients; however, valproic acid may be used as an alternative treatment.

IDIOPATHIC RECURRENT STUPOR

Idiopathic recurrent stupor, a rare condition, is characterized by recurrent episodes of stupor that occur without any metabolic, toxic, or structural brain dysfunctions. Episodes of stupor vary from one to six per year to more than six per year; durations of episodes range from 2 to 120 hours. Patients may be aroused briefly from the stupor. EEG shows nonreactive diffusely distributed fast rhythms

(14–16 Hz). Endozepine-4 in plasma and cerebrospinal fluid is markedly elevated in patients. After the administration of 0.5–1.5 mg intravenous flumazenil, a benzodiazepine-receptor antagonist, clinical manifestations and EEG abnormalities are rapidly reversed to their normal states.

FATAL FAMILIAL INSOMNIA

Fatal familial insomnia (FFI) is a rare autosomal-dominant prion disease with a mutation at codon 178 of the prion protein gene (PrP). Clinical manifestations of this disease include impaired control of the sleep–wake cycle (e.g., circadian rhythm, autonomic, and neuroendocrine dysfunction), in addition to somatic neurologic, cognitive, and behavioral manifestations. From the onset of illness, profound sleep disturbances (particularly severe insomnia) are noted. Ataxia, corticospinal deficit, myoclonus, and tremor are the characteristic neurologic deficits that occur in FFI. The condition runs a rapid, progressive course of 7–48 months, with an average duration of 12 months. PSG study shows an almost total absence of sleep pattern; only short episodes of REM sleep exist, lasting for a few seconds or minutes without the muscle atonia associated with dream-enacting behavior that occurs as complex movements and gestures (i.e., RBD). Characteristic neuropathologic findings consist of severe atrophy of the thalamus (especially anterior ventral and dorsomedial thalamic nuclei) associated with variable involvement of the inferior olive, striatum, and cerebellum.

LABORATORY INVESTIGATIONS

Laboratory tests should be conducted as an extension of patient histories and physical examinations. Tests should be directed at diagnosing primary neurologic disorders and assessing sleep disturbances that result from neurologic illnesses. (Refer to neurologic texts for details of neurodiagnostic tests to assess neurologic conditions responsible for sleep disorders.) Tests to assess primary neurologic disorders include neurophysiologic tests (EEG, electromyography, and evoked potentials); neuroimaging studies (computed tomography, magnetic resonance imaging, single-photon emission computed tomography, and positron emission tomography); examination of cerebrospinal fluid; and general laboratory tests, including blood work and urinalysis. Special procedures, such as tests to uncover autonomic deficits, neuroimmunologic, neurovirologic, or neurourologic investigations, and brain biopsies, are required to detect some neurologic disorders.

LABORATORY TESTS TO ASSESS SLEEP DISTURBANCE

Laboratory tests used to investigate sleep and sleep-related breathing disorders in neurologic illnesses include overnight PSG recording, MSLT, maintenance of wakefulness test, actigraphy, video-PSG, long-term video-EEG monitoring, and EEG including 24-hour EEG (see Chapter 7). Other tests include intracranial recordings conducted in specialized epilepsy centers for identifying seizure foci in patients with epilepsy and pulmonary function tests to exclude intrinsic bronchopulmonary disease, which may affect sleep-related breathing disorders.

MANAGEMENT OF SLEEP DISTURBANCES IN NEUROLOGIC DISORDERS

To manage sleep disturbances in neurologic disorders, accurate diagnoses of primary neurologic disorders must first occur. Diagnosis is followed by vigorous treatment and monitoring of the neurologic illness. Treatment of secondary sleep disturbances is unlikely to be successful unless primary causes are properly diagnosed and treated. Treatment of underlying causes may improve sleep disturbances. If a satisfactory treatment is not available for a primary condition or does not resolve the problem, however, treatment should be directed to the specific sleep disturbance. Readers are referred to neurologic texts for treatments of primary neurologic conditions.

Sleep disturbances occurring in neurologic disorders include hypersomnia, insomnia, circadian rhythm sleep disorders, and parasomnias. Treatments for these complaints are discussed in Chapters 10, 11, 12, 17, and 18. Treatment of hypersomnia resulting mainly from sleep-related respiratory dysrhythmias in neurologic disorders is briefly discussed below. General principles of treatment for sleep in AD and related dementias is reviewed in the section Treatment of Sleep in Alzheimer's Disease and Related Dementias.

The objective of treating sleep-related breathing disorders is improving quality of life by improving quality of sleep and preventing life-

Table 14.6
Treatment of sleep-related respiratory dysrhythmias in neurologic illnesses

---

General measures
Pharmacologic agents
Mechanical devices
    Nasal continuous positive airway pressure
    Other ventilatory supports
Supplemental oxygen therapy
Surgical measures

---

threatening cardiac arrhythmias, pulmonary hypertension, and congestive heart failure, each related to sleep-disordered breathing. Treatment modalities for sleep-related respiratory dysrhythmias resulting from neurologic illness can be divided into five categories (see Chapter 10): general measures, pharmacologic agents, mechanical devices, supplemental oxygen administration, and surgical treatment (Table 14.6).

General measures and pharmacologic treatments have been briefly reviewed in Chapter 10.

Mechanical Devices

Nasal Continuous Positive Airway Pressure

Nasal continuous positive airway pressure (CPAP) is an important therapeutic advance in the treatment of obstructive sleep apnea syndrome (OSAS) and has been described in Chapter 10. Nasal CPAP should be given a trial in patients with neurologic disorders who experience upper airway OSAS associated with intermittent central sleep or mixed apneas. Such treatment often improves quality of sleep and reduces daytime symptoms by eliminating or reducing sleep-related obstructive or mixed apneas and oxygen desaturation. Instead of CPAP, some patients may require bilevel positive airway pressure, which delivers a higher pressure during inspiration than during expiration. The role of nasal CPAP in central sleep apnea (CSA) syndrome is highly controversial. In a subgroup of patients with CSA who show narrowing or occlusion of the upper airway on fiberoptic scope, nasal CPAP may reverse apneic episodes.

Other Ventilatory Supports

In patients with neuromuscular disorders, including those with ALS, poliomyelitis, and postpolio syndrome, ventilatory support with either negative-pressure or positive-pressure ventilators is often required. Intermittent positive-pressure ventilation (IPPV) can be administered through a nasal mask. Negative-pressure ventilation can be delivered from a tank respirator or from a cuirass. With ventilatory support, patients with neuromuscular disorders tend to experience relief of daytime hypersomnolence with improvement of sleep architecture. In some patients, a combination of nasal mask and positive-pressure ventilation may be needed. When OSAS complicates sleep hypoventilation, IPPV through a nasal mask during sleep may be a better treatment than negative-pressure ventilation and may obviate the need for tracheostomy or diaphragm pacing. Negative-pressure ventilation may improve patients' nocturnal ventilation during NREM sleep, but can produce upper airway obstructive apnea during REM sleep, causing severe hypoxemia and hypercapnia. A combination of CPAP, cuirass, and, later, IPPV at night may be required in patients with respiratory muscle weakness (including diaphragmatic muscle weakness). Patients with motor neuron disease and associated sleep-related hypoventilation and apnea have been treated with this combination with considerable symptomatic relief. Patients with poliomyelitis or postpolio syndrome who require ventilatory support to maintain respiratory homeostasis generally show improvement in sleep architecture and respiratory function after mechanical ventilation via nasal mask. Those with obstructive or mixed apneas respond to CPAP.

Supplemental Oxygen Therapy

Supplemental oxygen therapy may decrease severity of OSAS in certain patients. Recommended treatment for nocturnal hypoxemia is administration of oxygen at a low flow rate (1–2 liters per minute) via a nasal cannula. Oxygen administration may not be safe for all patients. For neuromuscular patients with oxygen-sensitive hypoventilation, nocturnal assisted ventilation should be considered. In such patients, it may be possible to safely administer oxygen during the daytime.

Surgical Treatment

In patients with respiratory center involvement with CSA syndrome, diaphragm pacing and electrophrenic respiration have been used successfully, particularly in those patients who require ventilatory assistance during the day and night.

Tracheostomy has largely been replaced by CPAP titration, but may still be required occasionally as an emergency measure in patients who experience severe respiratory compromise or severe apnea associated

Table 14.7
Treatment of sleep disturbances in patients with Alzheimer's disease
and related dementias

Institute regular sleep schedule as much as possible
Eliminate alcohol and caffeine in the evening
Try an intermediate-acting benzodiazepine or zolpidem for no longer than
   three times/wk to treat insomnia
Reduce or eliminate medications that may contribute to sleep disturbances
   or sleep-related respiratory dysrhythmias
Treat associated depression with a sedative antidepressant
Treat associated conditions that may interfere with sleep (e.g., pain caused
   by arthritis and other causes)
Discourage patients from taking daytime naps
Encourage regular exercise (e.g., walking)
For extreme agitation, use small doses of haloperidol (0.5–1.0 mg BID or TID)
   or thioridazine (25 mg TID)
In selected patients, use bright light therapy in the evening

---

with dangerous cardiac arrhythmias, which cause life-threatening situations. Such patients may later be weaned.

TREATMENT OF SLEEP DISTURBANCES IN ALZHEIMER'S DISEASE AND RELATED DEMENTIAS

Table 14.7 lists general principles of treatment for sleep disturbances in patients with AD or related dementias. Medication that may have an adverse effect on sleep and breathing may be changed or reduced in dose. Associated pain due to arthritis and other causes that may interfere with sleep should be treated with analgesics. Depression is often an important feature in patients with AD; therefore, sedative-antidepressants may be helpful. Frequency of urination in such patients may result from infection or enlarged prostate, and may disturb sleep at night. Appropriate measures should be taken in such conditions. Patients should be encouraged to develop good sleep habits. Patients should avoid daytime naps and should be encouraged to exercise (e.g., walk during the day). They should not drink caffeinated beverages before bedtime or in the evening. For sleeplessness, a trial with intermediate-acting benzodiazepines or zolpidem should be conducted for a short period. Haloperidol should be tried for extreme agitation and confusion. In some patients, timed exposure to bright light in the evening may improve nighttime sleep.

15

Sleep in Psychiatric Disorders

Sleep disturbances are common in psychiatric disorders, with insomnia noted more commonly than hypersomnia in patients. The increased prevalence of sleep disorders occurring in patients with psychiatric illnesses and subsequent occurrence of psychiatric disorders in patients with sleep disorders (particularly those patients with insomnia) have been verified in a number of surveys. A large epidemiologic study found that individuals with insomnia at baseline were 34 times more likely than individuals without insomnia to develop a new psychiatric disorder within a year, particularly major depression. In addition, individuals with insomnia that is resolved within a year have similar incidence of subsequent psychiatric disorders. Specific examples of psychiatric conditions that are associated with insomnia include depression (including bipolar disorder), anxiety disorders, schizophrenia, and post-traumatic stress disorder. Hypersomnia is generally present in patients with seasonal affective disorder and may also be present in some cases of major depression.

AFFECTIVE DISORDERS

Depression is highly prevalent among elderly individuals who experience insomnia. Early morning awakening, although not a specific symptom of depression, is thought to be a hallmark of it in older individuals. Adolescents and young adults with depression may report difficulty initiating sleep. Insomnia is noted in approximately 90% of cases of major depression; excessive daytime somnolence (EDS) is found in a small percentage of patients, particularly in young adults. Characteristic polysomnographic (PSG) findings in depression include short rapid eye movement (REM) sleep latency; maldistribution of REM cycle duration, with the longest nocturnal REM cycle occurring in the first one-third of the night (instead of the last one-third of the night, as noted in individuals with normal sleep); and increased REM density (i.e., increased number of phasic REMs per minute of sleep). Early investigations suggested that REM sleep abnormality was a biological marker for depression; however, later investigations proved that this finding was nonspecific and REM sleep abnormality may also be noted in other psychiatric conditions. Other PSG findings include reduced sleep efficiency, decreased slow wave sleep (SWS), and a shift of SWS from the first nonrapid eye movement (NREM) cycle to the second cycle. Another microarchitectural finding described as occurring in depression is high amplitude fast frequency electroencephalography.

Although insomnia (particularly early morning awakening) is a characteristic of depression, some patients with major depression, especially those patients with bipolar depression, may experience hypersomnolence rather than insomnia. Individuals with seasonal affective disorder (SAD) with recurrent episodes of depression during winter months (i.e., "winter depression") more often have hypersomnolence rather than insomnia.

ANXIETY DISORDERS

Anxiety disorders are the most common psychiatric disorders and include generalized anxiety disorder, as well as panic, phobic, obsessive-compulsive, and post-traumatic stress disorders. Characteristic PSG findings in anxiety disorders include prolonged sleep-onset latency, reduced SWS and REM sleep (but increased stage I and stage II NREM sleep), and normal or increased REM latency.

Panic disorder patients generally experience panic attacks during the daytime, but some panic attacks occur at night. Symptoms of panic attacks are marked anxiety and fear associated with autonomic symptoms such as hyperventilation, palpitation, trembling, increased heart rate, sweating, flushing, and fear of imminent death. Major depression coexists with generalized anxiety and panic disorders in many patients. Sleep-related panic attacks resembling night terrors may disrupt sleep; these attacks usually occur during the transition from stage II NREM sleep to SWS but sometimes may arise from REM sleep. On awakening from sleep attacks, patients with panic attacks have clear memories of the spells, in contrast to those patients who experience night terrors, who do not have clear memories.

In patients with obsessive-compulsive disorder (OCD), obsessions and compulsions may cause severe anxiety, interfering with sleep. PSG findings in OCD include reduced sleep efficiency, increased awakenings, reduced SWS, and shortened REM latency.

Post-traumatic stress disorder (PTSD) is characterized by preoccupation with and the re-enactment of severely traumatic or life-threatening past events such as war experience, torture, or other situations involving physical or sexual abuse. Symptoms include flashbacks and anxiety-prone dreams. Patients with PTSD experience chronic insomnia owing to states of hyperarousal. PSG findings in PTSD include decreased total sleep time, reduced SWS and REM sleep, an increased number of awakenings, and impaired sleep efficiency. Frequent nightmares that may occur during NREM and REM sleep are hallmarks of PTSD. REM sleep findings in PTSD are contradictory. Some reports find reduced REM latency whereas others report prolonged REM latency. Some experts consider PTSD a disorder of the REM sleep mechanism and associate it with REM sleep behavior disorder.

SCHIZOPHRENIA

In schizophrenia, severity of sleep disturbance is related to intensity of psychotic symptoms. Often, an extremely prolonged sleep-onset latency during acute illness with reduction of total sleep time occurs. PSG findings in schizophrenia have been somewhat contradictory; reduced sleep efficiency and increased sleep latency in schizophrenia are the most consistent findings. REM sleep findings have been variable; reduced and normal REM latencies have been reported. In most studies, SWS is decreased. One difference between acute and chronic schizophrenic patients in terms of REM sleep abnormalities is the absence of REM sleep rebound after REM sleep deprivation in acute schizophrenics, in contrast with increased REM sleep rebound in chronic schizophrenics.

EATING DISORDERS

Patients with eating disorders may have significant sleep complaints. Weight loss, which occurs in anorexia nervosa, is associated with insomnia, whereas weight gain, which occurs in bulimia nervosa, is associated with hypersomnia. Many patients with eating disorders experience major depression, a condition that may be responsible for prominent sleep complaints in many of these patients. Findings of REM sleep abnormalities in eating disorders have been contradictory.

SLEEP DISORDERS AS A RESULT OF MEDICATIONS USED TO TREAT PSYCHIATRIC DISORDERS

Antidepressants, such as tricyclics, monoamine oxidase (MAO) inhibitors, and others (e.g., trazodone, fluoxetine, bupropion, ritanserin, and lithium), may cause sleep disruption, altered sleep architecture, and may suppress REM sleep. Sedative antidepressants (e.g., amitriptyline [Elavil], doxepin, and trazodone) may be used to treat insomnia, especially if it is associated with depression. Most tricyclic antidepressants may cause daytime sedation. Because MAO inhibitors have alerting properties, they should be used in the morning or early afternoon. Trazodone, a sedative antidepressant, increases SWS but is a weak REM suppressant. Fluoxetine has an alerting effect and can suppress REM sleep at high doses. Lithium increases SWS and has a mild REM suppressant effect. Sudden withdrawal of these REM-suppressing medications may cause REM rebound.

Neuroleptics, such as haloperidol, phenothiazine, and thioridazine, are used to treat schizophrenia and other psychotic conditions. Some of these drugs, particularly phenothiazine, may cause drowsiness and impair performance. All neuroleptics may produce serious side effects in combination with hypnotics, alcohol, or antihistaminic agents.

Alcohol has profound effects on sleep–wakefulness and is often abused by patients with psychiatric disorders. Acute administration of alcohol, a central nervous system sedative, causes reduced sleep onset, increased SWS, and reduced REM sleep. However, after initial sedative effects diminish and as the blood alcohol level falls, patients experience repeated awakenings, causing sleep fragmentation and REM rebound. (REM rebound is also noted on discontinuation after several nights of alcohol consumption.) The sedative action of alcohol may be caused by its facilitation of γ–aminobutyric acid function and inhibition of glutamate. Alcohol, barbiturates, and tricyclic antidepressants may also produce REM sleep behavior disorder and other state dissociations.

ASSESSMENT AND TREATMENT OF SLEEP DISORDERS IN PSYCHIATRIC CONDITIONS

Assessment of sleep disturbances in psychiatric patients should follow the general guidelines discussed in Chapter 7. A detailed sleep history, including any history that suggests an underlying sleep disorder other than psychiatric illness exists, should be obtained. It may be important to refer the patient to a psychiatrist for correct psychiatric assessment and diagnosis. Psychological tests (e.g., Minnesota Multiphasic Personality Inventory, Beck Depression Inventory, or Hamilton depression score) may be useful for screening patients but are limited in terms of diagnosis.

Primary psychiatric illnesses should be first treated with appropriate medications. Insomnia in major depression may be treated with a sedative antidepressant (e.g., tricyclics or trazodone). Sometimes, in addition to antidepressants, sedatives may be prescribed. Selective serotonin-reuptake inhibitors (SSRIs) may be combined with other sedative antidepressants (like trazodone) to improve a patient's sleep. Drug interactions may be a serious problem in such situations, in addition to patients' developing the "serotonin syndrome." Behavioral techniques have been found to be useful in improving insomnia in patients with psychiatric illness.

Schizophrenic patients require sedative neuroleptics for treatment of severe sleep disturbance and sometimes may require additional sedative-hypnotics.

Generalized anxiety disorders should be treated with a combination of behavioral techniques, or in severe cases, benzodiazepines or tricyclics. Patients with panic disorders respond best to benzodiazepines (such as alprazolam) or SSRIs. Sleep disorders associated with phobic anxiety should be treated with a combination of sleep restriction and benzodiazepine. Treatment of OCD consists of a combination of psychotherapy or behavioral therapy and drugs such as MAO inhibitors, tricyclics, or fluoxetine (Prozac). Similarly, eating disorders should be treated with a combination of psychotherapy and drug therapy, and many patients respond satisfactorily to fluoxetine (Prozac). Treatment for PTSD consists of psychotherapy, tricyclic antidepressants, MAO inhibitors, and, sometimes, lithium. SAD can be treated by bright light exposure in the morning. Those SAD patients who awake during early morning hours should be treated with bright light exposure in the evening. Adjunctive treatments include tricyclic antidepressants, MAOs, and lithium.

16

Sleep Disturbances in Other Medical Disorders

The International Classification of Sleep Disorders lists seven medical disorders associated with sleep disturbances: (1) nocturnal cardiac ischemia, (2) chronic obstructive pulmonary disease (COPD), (3) sleep-related asthma, (4) sleep-related gastroesophageal reflux, (5) peptic ulcer disease, (6) fibromyalgia, and (7) sleeping sickness. A number of other medical disorders exist, however, that may cause severe disturbances of sleep and breathing and have important practical implications in terms of diagnosis, prognosis, and treatment. These other medical disorders, which are not listed in the International Classification of Sleep Disorders, are included in this chapter because sleep disturbances may adversely affect their courses, and these medical disorders, as well as the drugs prescribed to treat them, may have deleterious effects on sleep and breathing.

GENERAL SLEEP COMPLAINTS AND MECHANISMS OF SLEEP DISTURBANCES IN MEDICAL DISORDERS

Most patients with medical disorders present with insomnia but some may present with a mixture of insomnia and hypersomnolence (e.g., patients with COPD, nocturnal asthma, nocturnal angina, and some endocrine diseases). Table 16.1 lists general medical causes of hypersomnia. The general medical causes of insomnia are listed in Table 11.3.

General medical disorders may affect sleep–wake neurons by indirect mechanisms through metabolic, toxic, or anoxic disturbances. Furthermore, sleep-related breathing disturbances in general medical disorders may affect sleep profoundly, causing sleep apnea–hypopnea, fragmentation of sleep, and daytime hypersomnolence. Medications

Table 16.1
General medical causes of hypersomnia

Hepatic, renal, or respiratory failure
Electrolyte disturbances
Congestive cardiac failure
Severe anemia
Endocrine diseases (hypothyroidism, acromegaly, Addison's disease)
Diabetes mellitus (hypoglycemia, hyperglycemia)

---

used to treat medical disorders may also affect sleep and breathing. Sleep–wake schedule disturbances and associated depression, anxiety, and alterations of the chemical environment are other factors that disrupt sleep in these disorders.

SPECIFIC MEDICAL DISORDERS AND SLEEP DISTURBANCES

Ischemic Heart Disease and Nocturnal Angina

Sleep-related profound hemodynamic changes (e.g., unstable blood pressure and heart rate during REM sleep, or the reduction of cardiac output during rapid eye movement [REM] and nonrapid eye movement [NREM] sleep) and sympathetic alterations (which decrease with intermittent increases in REM sleep) may trigger thrombotic events, causing myocardial infarction, ventricular arrhythmias, or even sudden cardiac death. Adequate objective tests for documenting sleep disturbances and other catastrophic cardiovascular events—including polysomnographic (PSG) study—are lacking, however. An enhanced parasympathetic tone during sleep tends to confer an antiarrhythmic effect on ventricular premature beats. Ventricular arrhythmias, however, have been reported to occur during arousal from sleep as a result of increased sympathetic activity.

A variety of sleep disturbances are described in patients admitted to intensive care units with acute myocardial infarctions; these include decreased sleep efficiency, increased sleep stage shifts, increased awakenings, and decreased REM sleep on PSG study. Autonomic denervation may contribute to the development of ventricular tachyarrhythmias. Nocturnal anginal pain may awaken patients, causing impaired sleep efficiency and frequent awakenings.

Congestive Cardiac Failure

Cheyne-Stokes respiration, commonly associated with congestive cardiac failure, may cause hypoxemia, hypercapnia, sleep disruption owing to repeated arousals, excessive daytime somnolence (EDS), and impaired cognitive function. Cheyne-Stokes breathing in congestive cardiac failure may, in fact, present as sleep apnea syndrome. Patients may benefit from treatment with continuous positive airway pressure (CPAP) titration and nocturnal oxygen administration. The role of CPAP in central apnea of heart failure is not clear.

Systemic Hypertension

A high prevalence (22–48%) of sleep apnea and related symptoms exists in patients with systemic hypertension. Although controversial, evidence that obstructive sleep apnea syndrome (OSAS) may be an independent risk factor exists, and treatment of OSAS may reduce daytime and nighttime blood pressure.

Chronic Obstructive Pulmonary Disease

In patients with COPD (e.g., chronic bronchitis and emphysema), blood gases show a rise in partial pressure of carbon dioxide in arterial gas and fall in partial pressure of arterial oxygen and oxygen saturation during sleep, with worsening occurring during REM sleep. Alveolar hypoventilation, worse during REM sleep, and ventilation-profusion mismatching are important factors affecting worsening hypoxemia during sleep. When COPD coexists with OSAS, the condition is known as *overlap syndrome*. Sleep architectural changes in COPD patients include a reduction in sleep efficiency, delayed sleep onset, increased awakenings, frequent stage shifts, and arousals. An increased prevalence of cardiac arrhythmias exists in COPD patients, particularly during sleep. Nocturnal hypoxemia in COPD patients may be effectively treated by administering low-flow oxygen at a rate of 1–2 liters per minute. A number of factors may be responsible for sleep disturbance in COPD patients, including drugs used to treat the condition (e.g., methylxanthine, causing insomnia) or increased nocturnal cough with an accumulation of bronchial secretions, associated with hypoxemia and hypercapnia.

Bronchial Asthma

Sleep disturbances occurring in bronchial asthma (including those occurring in nocturnal asthma) consist of a combination of insomnia and hypersomnia, with difficulties in maintaining sleep, early morning awakenings, and EDS. Progressive bronchoconstriction and hypoxemia occurring during sleep in patients with asthma cause nocturnal exacerbations of symptoms. PSG study may document loss of total sleep time, frequent awakenings, reduced slow wave sleep (SWS), and sleep apnea in some of these patients. Autonomic dysfunction and circadian factors have been cited as pathogenetic mechanisms for sleep disturbances with nocturnal exacerbations of asthma.

Peptic Ulcer Disease

Patients with peptic ulcer disease may have repeated arousals and awakenings as a result of episodes of nocturnal epigastric pain. A characteristic observation in duodenal ulcer patients is the occurrence of a failure to inhibit gastric acid secretion during the first 2 hours after sleep onset.

Gastroesophageal Reflux Disease

Reflux esophagitis or gastroesophageal reflux disease (GERD) may cause difficulty in initiating sleep, frequent awakenings, and fragmentation of sleep related to symptoms of retrosternal burning pain owing to repeated spontaneous reflux episodes. A potential complication of repeated reflux episodes is Barrett's esophagus, a disorder that may be a precursor to esophageal adenocarcinoma. Sleep itself affects patients with GERD by increasing episodes of reflux and prolonging acid clearance time. Such reflux episodes may also exacerbate asthmatic attacks in patients with nocturnal asthma.

Endocrine Diseases

Upper airway obstructive and central sleep apneas, related to a deposition of mucopolysaccharides in the upper airway and impaired central respiratory drive, have been described in many patients with myxedema.

Central sleep apnea causing sleep disturbances has been noted in association with the pituitary gland's growth-hormone release in patients with acromegaly. Such patients may respond to treatment with octreotide, a long-acting somatostatin analog.

In patients with diabetes mellitus, especially those cases associated with autonomic neuropathy, central and obstructive sleep apneas causing EDS and sleep fragmentation have been described.

Chronic Renal Failure

In chronic renal failure (CRF) patients, insomnia, EDS, and disturbed nocturnal sleep with reversed day and night sleep rhythms are common sleep complaints. PSG study shows reduced sleep efficiency, increased sleep fragmentation, frequent awakenings with difficulty in maintenance of sleep, and decreased SWS. Restless legs syndrome (RLS) and periodic limb movements in sleep (PLMS) are common in uremic patients. Uremic RLS and idiopathic RLS resemble each other and cannot be distinguished clinically. One report of a cure for this form of RLS, achieved after successful kidney transplantation, exists. Many CRF patients also experience sleep apnea syndrome, mainly obstructive in nature, on and off dialysis.

Sleep–Wake Disturbances in Intensive Care Unit Patients

Patients with acute medical, surgical, and neurologic disorders are admitted to the intensive care unit (ICU), where comorbid conditions are responsible for severe sleep disturbances such as insomnia, hypersomnia, and sleep-related respiratory dysrhythmias. Other factors contributing to sleep disturbances in the ICU include environment (e.g., noise, bright light, and constant activity in the unit due to monitoring and drug administration), sleep deprivation, and a variety of drugs used to treat ICU patients. ICU syndrome is characterized by a typical mental state (defined as a reversible confusional state) that develops 3–7 days after ICU admission and is secondary to sleep deprivation. Some ICU patients may experience REM sleep behavior disorder (RBD). PSG study may show diminished SWS and REM sleep, frequent awakenings, and reduced total sleep time. ICU patients often acquire EDS as a result of night-sleep disturbance. Awareness of the various ICU factors that contribute to sleep disturbance is important so that correct diagnoses can be made and management of secondary complications, in addition to treatment of primary disorders, can be instituted promptly. Both nonpharmacologic and pharmacologic interventions are required for treatment of sleep disturbances in the ICU.

Acquired Immunodeficiency Syndrome

Acquired immunodeficiency syndrome (AIDS), caused by the human immunodeficiency virus type 1 (HIV-1) is a systemic disease affecting different body systems through opportunistic infections and associated neoplasms. Neurologic manifestations occur in almost half of all AIDS patients and include HIV encephalopathy, myelopathy, peripheral neuropathy, and polyradiculopathy. Sleep disturbances have been reported in many patients as a manifestation of encephalopathy, which may also cause seizures, dementia, and focal or diffuse central nervous system (CNS) dysfunctions. Sleep dysfunctions include sleep apnea with sleep fragmentation and EDS, sleep initiation, and maintenance difficulties. Some reports of sleep dysfunction based on questionnaires and PSG studies in seropositive patients in absence of full-blown AIDS exist. Involvement of sleep–wake neurons in the brain stem and hypothalamic-preoptic region is presumed to be responsible for sleep abnormalities in AIDS. A systematic study of a large number of patients (including PSG study) is required to comprehend the prevalence of sleep disturbances that exist in AIDS and also to find out if PSG can document specific sleep abnormalities in asymptomatic individuals.

Lyme Disease

Lyme disease is a multisystem disease caused by *Borrelia burgdorferi*, transmitted to humans via tick bites. Sleep complaints are common in Lyme disease and PSG findings include decreased sleep efficiency, increased arousal index with sleep fragmentation, and alpha intrusion into NREM sleep. Sleep complaints consist of difficulty initiating sleep, frequent awakenings, and EDS, as well as fatigue.

Chronic Fatigue Syndrome

Chronic fatigue syndrome is an ill-defined heterogeneous condition. One major diagnostic criterion is an insidious onset of fatigue occurring for at least 6 months without any evident causes (despite extensive laboratory investigations). Minor criteria include arthralgias, myalgias, headaches, and sleep disturbances. The cause of chronic fatigue syndrome remains undetermined. A tilt table study documented orthostatic hypotension in several patients, but the significance and prevalence of orthostatic hypotension in chronic fatigue syndrome cannot be determined without further systematic study of a large number of patients from different centers. Sleep disturbances have not been well characterized. In isolated reports, complaints of disturbed night sleep and EDS exist. A few PSG studies have shown coexistent primary sleep disorders such as sleep apnea, PLMS, and narcolepsy.

Hematologic Disorders

Paroxysmal nocturnal hemoglobinuria may cause sleep disturbance associated with increased levels of plasma hemoglobin in the middle of the night and early hours of the morning. Obstructive sleep apnea and reduced arterial oxygen saturation during sleep, causing sleep disturbance, have been described in patients with sickle cell anemia. Hereditary hemorrhagic telangiectasia may cause progressive somnolence accompanied by confusion.

Fibromyalgia Syndrome

Fibromyalgia syndrome (FMS) is characterized by diffuse muscle aches and pains not related to diseases of the joints, bones, or connective tissues; it presents with multiple tender spots. The neck and shoulder joints and sacrospinal and gluteal regions are common sites of these aches and pains. Specific diagnostic criteria have been established. Differential diagnoses include polymyalgia rheumatica, chronic fatigue syndrome, and other myofacial pain syndromes. Its cause remains undetermined. Sleep disturbance is common in FMS. A characteristic PSG finding is intermittent alpha intrusion into NREM sleep, giving rise to characteristic alpha-delta or alpha-NREM sleep anomaly. Alpha-NREM sleep is not specific for FMS, as it has also been described in other rheumatic and psychiatric disorders, post-viral fatigue syndrome, febrile illness, and even in individuals without specific medical conditions. Alpha-NREM sleep, however, has been noted more frequently in FMS than in any other condition. The most prominent complaint in patients with FMS is nonrestorative sleep associated with nonspecific PSG findings of sleep fragmentation, increased awakenings, and decreased sleep efficiency. Treatment of this condition has been unsatisfactory and consists of pharmacologic therapy with tricyclic antidepressants, short-term intermittent treatment with zolpidem, exercise programs, education, and reassurance.

Dermatologic Disorders

Painful skin diseases and nighttime pruritus may cause sleep-initiating and maintenance insomnia. Recurrent episodes of pruritus, noted most frequently during stages I and II NREM sleep and least frequently in SWS, have been noted in some dermatologic disorders.

African Sleeping Sickness

African sleeping sickness, or trypanosomiasis, is caused by *Trypanosoma gambiense* or *Trypanosoma rhodesiense* and is transmitted to humans via the bites of Tsetse flies. Circadian rhythm disruption with reversal of the sleep–wake rhythm is the most prominent finding. Patients remain somnolent in the daytime and gradually progress into stages of stupor or coma. In the most advanced stages, a circadian disruption of plasma cortisol and prolactin along with disruptions of sleep–wake rhythms are noted, findings that suggest selective changes in the suprachiasmatic nuclei occur. Diagnosis is based on history and confirmation of the organism in the blood, bone marrow, cerebrospinal fluid, lymph node aspirates, and chancre scrapings.

Other Medical Conditions Causing Sleep Disturbance

Hepatic encephalopathy and severe electrolyte disturbances may cause hypersomnolence, asterixis, and multifocal myoclonus. Severe anemia

Table 16.2
Painful medical conditions causing insomnia

Anginal pain
Peptic ulcer pain
Pain associated with systemic cancer
Renal pain
Rheumatic diseases
Nocturnal pruritus
Nocturnal cramps

---

may cause hypersomnia; painful medical disorders may cause insomnia (Table 16.2). PSG findings in patients with pain show increased sleep latency, wakefulness after sleep onset, and arousal, and reduced SWS and alpha-NREM anomaly. Associated conditions, such as depression, anxiety, and PLMS, also aggravate sleep disturbance in painful conditions.

Medication-Related Sleep–Wake Disturbances

Medications used to treat general medical disorders may cause either sleepiness or insomnia (Table 16.3). Antihistamines (H_1 blockers) used to treat allergies cause drowsiness and daytime sleepiness. Narcotics (morphine, codeine, and other opioids) used to treat severe pain can cause CNS sedation. Aspirin may also have a mild hypnotic effect. Antiemetics (metoclopramide, domperidone, phenothiazines, and anticholinergic scopolamine) may cause drowsiness. Angiotensin-converting enzyme inhibitors used to treat hypertension may affect sleep adversely, causing impairment of performance and mood. Beta blockers (propranolol, metoprolol, and pindolol) used to treat hypertension, cardiac arrhythmias, and angina may cause difficulty in initiating sleep and increased awakenings or frequent nightmares. Bronchodilators and theophylline, used to treat COPD and bronchial asthma, may cause insomnia. Anorectics (appetite suppressants) increase catecholaminergic activity and act as CNS stimulants, causing insomnia. Sleeping pills, particularly long-acting ones, may affect daytime function. Short-acting hypnotic drugs may cause rebound insomnia, daytime anxiety, and amnesia. All hypnotics have respiratory depressant effects, particularly in patients with COPD, bronchial asthma, and sleep apnea. Sleeping medications should be used cautiously in the elderly, as these may easily induce side effects because metabolism and drug absorption are altered in elderly patients.

Table 16.3
Medications used in medical, neurologic, and psychiatric disorders causing
sleep disturbances

Medications causing sleepiness
  Antihistamines
  Narcotics
  Antiemetics
  Hypnotics
  Tricyclic antidepressants
  Neuroleptics
  Anticonvulsants
Medications causing insomnia
  Beta blockers
  Angiotensin-converting enzyme inhibitors
  Bronchodilators
  Corticosteroids
  Anorectics
  Nasal decongestants
  Amphetamines

Drugs used to treat psychiatric disorders, such as antidepressants, may cause sleep disruption, alter sleep architecture, and suppress REM sleep. Most tricyclic antidepressants may cause daytime sedation. Fluoxetine has an alerting effect and can suppress REM sleep at higher doses. Lithium increases SWS and has a mild REM-suppressant effect. Sudden withdrawal of REM suppressant medication may cause REM rebound. Neuroleptics may cause drowsiness and impair performance. All neuroleptics may produce serious side effects when combined with hypnotics, alcohol, or antihistaminic agents.

Over-the-counter medications, used as nasal decongestants and anorectics, are stimulants and cause insomnia. Caffeine, which is present in coffee, tea, colas, and chocolates, is a stimulant and may cause insomnia. Over-the-counter sleeping pills contain antihistamines (diphenhydramine and doxylamine) and may cause daytime sedation.

17

Circadian Regulation of Sleep and Circadian Sleep Disorders

Underlying rhythmicity is a fundamental property of all living organisms. The basic rest–activity cycle (i.e., the mammalian equivalent of the sleep–wakefulness cycle) present in all living matter is not only controlled by rhythmic geophysical fluctuations of light and darkness but also is an endogenous rhythm generated by an internal pacemaker or biological clock. The existence of circadian rhythms has been recognized since the eighteenth century when the French astronomer de Mairan noted a diurnal rhythm in heliotrope plants, which close their leaves at sunset and open them at sunrise—even when they are kept in darkness—shielding themselves from direct sunlight. This discovery of 24-hour rhythm in the movement of plant leaves suggested to de Mairan the existence of an internal clock in plants. Later experiments proved the existence of 24-hour rhythm in animals as well.

The term *circadian rhythm* is derived from the Lain *circa*, which means about, and *dien*, which means day (see Chapter 1). Rhythms with periods lasting shorter than a day are ultradian, those with periods lasting longer than a day (i.e., approximately a month) are infradian, and those approximately a year in length are circannual.

Experiments conducted in rats in 1972 clearly identified the site of a biological clock in the paired suprachiasmatic nuclei of the hypothalamus above the optic chiasm. Experimental stimulation, ablation, and lesion of these nuclei altered circadian rhythms. The existence of the suprachiasmatic nucleus (SCN) in humans was later confirmed. The SCN serves as a pacemaker, and its neurons are responsible for generating the circadian rhythms. Several neurotransmitters have been located within the terminals of the SCN, afferents, and interneurons, including serotonin, neuropeptide Y, vasopressin, vasoactive intestinal peptide, and γ-aminobutyric acid. The SCN has both afferent and efferent connections. The main afferent connection that exists is a direct retinohypothalamic tract from retinal ganglion cells, optic nerve, and optic chiasm to the small cluster of neurons in the SCN. An indirect afferent projection arises from the lateral geniculate nuclei, giving rise to the geniculohypothalamic tract. SCN also receives a robust serotonergic input from the midbrain raphe nuclei. Efferent projections from the SCN terminate in the paraventricular (PVN) and dorsomedial hypothalamic nuclei, thalamus, and pineal gland. The efferent pathway to the pineal gland begins as a projection from the SCN to the PVN that projects directly to the intermediolateral neurons of the spinal cord, which in turn project to the superior cervical ganglion, which, finally, provides sympathetic input to the pineal gland.

Circadian rhythm persists in free-running or constant environments when all external cues are removed (i.e., the rhythms are freed from environmental cues). This free-running rhythm can be phase-shifted by appropriately timed light pulses that occur during active periods. For example, bright light in the early morning phase-advances a rhythm, whereas bright light in the early evening phase-delays the rhythm. However, light exposure occurring in the middle of the day has no effect; this period is called *dead zone*. The concept of the phase response curve is based on research using bright light and indicates responses of advance, delay, or dead zone in activity cycles.

Daily rhythms are noted as occurring in several other human physiologic processes. Body temperature rhythm is sinusoidal, and cortisol and growth hormone secretion rhythms are pulsatile. It is well known that plasma levels of prolactin, growth hormone, and testosterone are all increased during sleep at night. Melatonin, the hormone synthesized from the pineal gland, is secreted maximally during the night and may be an important modulator of human circadian rhythm entrainment by the light–dark cycle. Sleep decreases body temperature, whereas activity and wakefulness increase it. Internal desynchronization occurs during free-running experiments, and body temperature rhythm dissociates from sleep rhythm as a result of that desynchronization. This observation raises the question of whether SCN is the master clock, or simply one of several clocks, existing in mammalian species.

Sleep and wakefulness are controlled by homeostatic and circadian factors (see Chapter 1).

CHRONOBIOLOGY, CHRONOPHARMACOLOGY, AND CHRONOTHERAPY

Chronobiology refers to the study of the body's biological responses to time-related events. All biological functions of cells, organs, and the entire body have circadian, ultradian, or infradian rhythms. It is important to remember that circadian timing may alter pathophysiologic responses in various disease states, resulting in events such as exacerbation of bronchial asthma at night, high incidence of stroke late at night, or myocardial infarction during early morning hours.

Chronopharmacology refers to biological responses to medications depending on the circadian timing of drug administration. Potential differences in responses of antibiotics to bacteria or of cancer cells to chemotherapy or radiotherapy, depending on times of administration, illustrate the importance of chronopharmacology.

Chronotherapy refers to the manipulation of circadian rhythms to treat certain circadian rhythm disorders (e.g., delayed and advanced sleep phase syndromes).

CIRCADIAN RHYTHM SLEEP DISORDERS

Circadian rhythm sleep disorders result from a mismatch between the body's internal clock and geophysical environment, either owing to malfunction of the biological clock (primary circadian rhythm disorders) or due to a shift in its environment that causes it to be out-of-phase (secondary circadian rhythm dysrhythmias). Table 17.1 lists the primary and secondary circadian rhythm disorders.

Jet Lag Syndrome

Jet lag is experienced as a result of eastward or westward jet travel, after travelers cross several time zones, disrupting synchronization between the body's inner clock and its external cues. Symptoms do not occur after north–south travel. Jet lag symptoms consist of difficulty in maintaining sleep, frequent arousals, and excessive daytime somno-

Table 17.1.
Classification of circadian rhythm sleep disorders

Primary circadian rhythm disorders
    Advanced sleep phase syndrome
    Delayed sleep phase syndrome
    Non–24-hour sleep–wake disorder
Secondary circadian rhythm disorders
    Jet lag
    Shift work sleep disorder
    Irregular sleep–wake disorder

---

lence. Symptoms of jet lag syndrome resolve within a few days to 2 weeks (see Chapter 11 for a more detailed discussion).

Treatment is unsatisfactory. Some investigators advocate the administration of 2–5 mg of melatonin 2 days before travel, at bedtime in the new time zone, with treatment continuing at bedtime in the new time zone for approximately 3 days. This schedule should be reversed when patients return to their original time zones. Other suggested treatment includes the administration of short-acting hypnotics (e.g., zolpidem) at the new bedtime, which may improve sleep and reduce some symptoms. Finally, exposure to appropriately timed sunlight may be helpful. After eastward travel, exposure to morning sunlight along with relative darkness in evening hours may facilitate adjustment. In contrast, for westward travel, evening light exposure may help shift the circadian clock.

Shift Work Sleep Disorder

Shift work sleep disorder may affect up to 5,000,000 workers in the United States and may include sleep disruption, chronic fatigue, and gastrointestinal symptoms (including peptic ulcer), increasing patients' chances of being involved in traffic accidents and making errors on the job. The symptoms of shift work sleep disorder rarely can be improved by adjusting to the work time schedule. For night shift workers, exposure to morning light on the way home may help keep the biological clock set to real world time. Melatonin has been found to be useful in some patients; however, research has not proven for certain whether melatonin alters the circadian phase or simply acts as a sedative to improve sleep.

Delayed Sleep Phase Syndrome

The International Classification of Sleep Disorders defines delayed sleep phase syndrome (DSPS) as a condition in which a patient's major sleep episode is delayed in relation to desired clock time. This delay causes symptoms of sleep-onset insomnia or difficulty awakening at the desired time. Typically, patients go to sleep late (e.g., between 2:00 AM and 6:00 AM) and awaken during late morning or afternoon hours (e.g., 10:00 AM to 2:00 PM). Patients with this disorder have great difficulties in functioning adequately during daytime hours if they must wake up early in the morning to go to school or work. These patients experience severe sleep onset difficulty; they cannot function normally in society due to disturbed sleep schedules. Patients often try a variety of hypnotic medications or alcohol in attempts to initiate sleep sooner.

Sleep architecture is generally normal if these individuals are allowed to follow their own uninterrupted sleep–wake schedule.

In some sleep disorders centers, DSPS may represent 5–10% of cases of patients complaining of insomnia. Onset generally occurs during childhood or adolescence. Sometimes, a history of DSPS in other family members exists. Some patients may experience depression. Primary DSPS may result from an unusually long intrinsic period owing to abnormality in the biological clock in the SCN. Actigraphic recordings and sleep logs kept over several days document characteristic sleep schedules.

DSPS patients may be treated profitably by the use of chronotherapy or phototherapy, or both. Chronotherapy is a therapy that intentionally delays sleep onset by 2–3 hours on successive days until a desired bedtime has been achieved. After a bedtime has been set, the patient strictly enforces the sleep–wake schedule. Some patients respond satisfactorily to this form of treatment, even when their disorder has been present for many years; after several months, however, many patients become less adherent to the schedule and begin to lapse into their original sleep habits.

Exposure to bright light on awakening is effective in altering sleep onset and synchronizing body temperature rhythms in patients with DSPS. Patients sit in front of a 10,000-lux light for 30–40 minutes on awakening. In addition, room lighting must be markedly reduced in the evening to achieve desired results. Response is generally evident after 2–3 weeks but frequently requires indefinite treatment to maintain. This treatment is still evolving. No large-scale study with adequate follow-up has been conducted.

Advanced Sleep Phase Syndrome

Advanced sleep phase syndrome (ASPS) is the converse of DSPS. Patients go to sleep in the early evening and wake up earlier than desired in the morning (e.g., 2:00–4:00 AM). Because these patients have early morning awakenings, they experience sleep disruption and daytime sleepiness if they do not go to sleep at early hours.

ASPS is most commonly seen in elderly individuals. Diagnosis is based on sleep logs and characteristic actigraphic recordings made over several days. The disorder is easy to distinguish from early awakenings in depression because sleep architecture is normal and does not exhibit the shortened rapid eye movement (REM) sleep latency and other REM sleep abnormalities seen in depressed patients. The basic mechanism thought to occur in DSPS is an inherent shortening of endogenous circadian timing. In some reports, a history of ASPS in other family members exists.

Chronotherapy may be used, gradually shifting a patient's time of sleep onset backward approximately 2–3 hours per day until sleep occurs at the desired time. Chronotherapy in ASPS is not as successful as in DSPS. Bright light exposure in the evening has been successful in delaying sleep onset.

Hypernychthemeral Syndrome

Hypernychthemeral syndrome, also known as *non–24-hour sleep–wake disorder*, is characterized by a patient's inability to maintain a regular bedtime and a sleep onset that occurs at irregular hours. Patients display increases in delay of sleep onset by approximately 1 hour per sleep–wake cycle, causing an eventual progression of sleep onset through the daytime hours and into the evening. These individuals fail to be entrained or synchronized by usual time cues such as sunlight or social activities.

This disorder is an extremely uncommon condition and is most often associated with blindness. Approximately one-third of blind individuals experience this disorder due to impairments of their retinohypothalamic pathway, which normally cues circadian patterns. This syndrome also may be associated with hypothalamic tumors. Sometimes depression and anxiety disorders are associated with this syndrome.

Melatonin (0.5–7.5 mg, taken orally in the evening or bedtime) has been reported to be effective in some blind persons who experience hypernychthemeral syndrome.

18

Parasomnias

Parasomnias can be defined as abnormal movements or behaviors that intrude into sleep intermittently or episodically during the night without generally disturbing sleep architecture. The International Classification of Sleep Disorders classifies parasomnias into four groups (see Table 7.1): (1) arousal disorders, (2) sleep–wake transition disorders, (3) rapid eye movement (REM)–related parasomnias, and (4) other parasomnias. This classification lists 24 distinct entities, several of which are rare. Major parasomnias can also be classified into motor and behavioral parasomnias. Motor parasomnias, abnormal movements intruding into sleep or an impairment of movements occurring during sleep, are classified into four categories (see Table 13.2): (1) nonrapid eye movement (NREM) sleep parasomnias, (2) REM sleep parasomnias, (3) sleep–wake transition disorders, and (4) diffuse parasomnias with no stage preferences. Several parasomnias occurring in NREM and rapid eye movement sleep may be mistaken for seizures (particularly, complex partial seizures). Somnambulism, night terror, confusional arousals, somniloquy, bruxism, rhythmic movement disorder, nocturnal enuresis, rapid eye movement sleep behavior disorder (RBD), and nightmares are some parasomnias that may be mistaken for seizures. RBD and nightmares are the only motor and behavioral parasomnias associated with REM sleep. Characteristic clinical features and electroencephalographic (EEG) and polysomnographic (PSG) recordings are essential in differentiating these conditions.

SOMNAMBULISM

Somnambulism, or sleepwalking, occurs most commonly in children between 5 and 12 years of age (Table 18.1). Sometimes, it persists into adulthood; rarely, it begins in adults. Sleepwalking begins with abrupt motor activity arising out of slow wave sleep (SWS) during the first

Table 18.1
Somnambulism (sleepwalking)

Onset: common between ages 5 and 12 yrs
High frequency of a positive family history
Abrupt onset of motor activity arising out of slow wave sleep during the first
  third of night
Duration: less than 10 mins
Injuries and violent activity: reported occasionally
Precipitating factors: sleep deprivation, fatigue, concurrent illness, sedatives
Treatment: precaution, benzodiazepines, imipramine

---

one-third of sleep. The episode generally lasts less than 10 minutes. A
high incidence of positive family history in sleepwalking exists. Injuries
and violent actions have been reported during sleepwalking episodes;
generally, however, individuals can negotiate their way around rooms.
Sleep deprivation, fatigue, concurrent illness, psychological stress, and
sedatives may act as precipitating factors.

SLEEP TERRORS

Sleep terrors, or *pavor nocturnus*, also occur during SWS (Table 18.2).
Peak onset occurs in children between 5 and 7 years of age. In sleep
terrors, as in sleepwalking, a high frequency of familial history exists.
Episodes of sleep terror are characterized by intense autonomic and
motor symptoms, including loud, piercing screams. Patients appear

Table 18.2
Sleep terror (*pavor nocturnus*)

Onset: peak occurs between ages 5 and 7 yrs
High frequency of familial cases
Abrupt arousal from slow wave sleep during the first third of night with
  loud, piercing scream
Intense autonomic and motor components
Many patients also sleepwalk
Precipitating factors: stress, sleep deprivation, fever
Treatment: psychotherapy, benzodiazepines, tricyclics

---

highly confused and fearful. Many patients also have histories of sleep-walking episodes. Precipitating factors are similar to those described in sleepwalking.

CONFUSIONAL AROUSALS

Confusional arousals occur mostly in children before age 5 years. As in sleepwalking and sleep terrors, these episodes arise with confusion out of SWS. Patients may exhibit automatic and inappropriate behavior, but the majority of spells that occur are benign, necessitating no treatment. Confusional arousals may be considered a mild form of sleep-walking and sleep terrors.

NIGHTMARES

Nightmares (also known as *dream anxiety attacks*) are fearful, vivid, and often frightening dreams that are mostly visual but sometimes auditory, seen during REM sleep. Nightmares may accompany sleep talk-ing and body movements, and most commonly occur during the middle to late part of sleep at night. Nightmares are mostly a normal phenomenon. At least 50% of children experience nightmares, begin-ning at ages 3–5 years. Frequencies of nightmares continuously decrease as children grow older, and elderly individuals have few or no nightmares. Frightening and recurrent nightmares (e.g., one or more nightmares per week) are not common and occur in less than 1% of individuals.

Nightmares can also occur as side effects of certain medications such as antiparkinsonian drugs (e.g., pergolide or levodopa), anticholiner-gics, and antihypertensive drugs (particularly beta blockers). Night-mares commonly occur after sudden withdrawal of REM-suppressant drugs (e.g., tricyclic antidepressants or selective serotonin reuptake inhibitors). Benzodiazepines (e.g., diazepam or clonazepam) often suppress nightmares; however, withdrawal from benzodiazepines may precipitate nightmares. Nightmares may also occur after alco-hol ingestion or sudden barbiturate withdrawal. Nightmares (along with severe sleep disturbance) may sometimes be initial manifesta-tions of schizophreniform psychosis. Many people with certain per-sonality types experience nightmares throughout life. Nightmares generally do not require any treatment except reassurance. In patients with recurring and fearful nightmares, however, combined

Table 18.3
Rapid eye movement sleep behavior disorder

Onset: occurs in middle-aged or elderly men
Presents with violent dream-enacting behavior during sleep, causing injury
   to self or bed partner
Often misdiagnosed as psychiatric disorder or nocturnal seizure (partial
   complex seizure)
Etiology: 55% idiopathic, 45% causal association with structural central
   nervous system lesion or related to alcohol or drugs (sedatives, hypnotics,
   tricyclics, anticholinergics)
Polysomnography: rapid eye movement sleep without muscle atonia
Experimental model: bilateral perilocus ceruleus lesions
Treatment: 90% respond to clonazepam

---

behavioral or psychotherapy and REM-suppressant medications may
be helpful.

RAPID EYE MOVEMENT SLEEP BEHAVIOR DISORDER

RBD is an important REM sleep parasomnia commonly observed in
elderly persons (Table 18.3). A characteristic feature of RBD is an
intermittent loss of REM-related muscle hypotonia or atonia, and
the appearance of various abnormal motor activities during sleep.
Patients experience violent dream-enacting behavior during REM
sleep, often causing self-injury or injury to bed partners. This condition may be either idiopathic or occur secondary to a neurologic
illness (e.g., Parkinson's disease, multiple system atrophy, olivopontocerebellar atrophy, and other structural lesions of the brain stem).
RBD is sometimes associated with alcoholism or ingestion of drugs
(e.g., sedative-hypnotics, tricyclic antidepressants, and anticholinergics). The most prominent finding in PSG recording of patients
who experience RBD is REM sleep without muscle atonia. Because
absence of muscle atonia may not be seen in all muscles, multiple
muscle electromyography (EMG) of the upper and lower extremities should be obtained during PSG recording, in addition to a traditional tibialis anterior muscle EMG. In experiments, similar
behaviors in cats were produced by bilateral perilocus ceruleus
lesions many years before discovery of human RBD.

ISOLATED SLEEP PARALYSIS

During sleep paralysis, an inability to perform voluntary movements, either at sleep onset (hypnagogic or predormital) or at sleep offset (hypnopompic or postdormital), occurs. Isolated sleep paralysis is much more common than is sleep paralysis as part of the narcolepsy–cataplexy syndrome tetrad. Subjects are conscious of environment and feel frightened and anxious due to apparent limb paralysis without affection of eye muscle or respiration. Episodes usually last for a few minutes and typically disappear, either spontaneously or when patients are touched by another person.

Forty percent to 50% of subjects with normal sleep functions experience isolated sleep paralysis at least once during their lifetimes. Onset generally occurs in young adults and adolescents, and both sexes are equally affected. A chronic familial form of sleep paralysis exists that affects females more often than males and has a sex-linked dominant transmission. Triggering factors often include sleep deprivation, psychological stress, and rotating shift work. PSG recordings have been obtained in sleep paralysis associated with narcolepsy–cataplexy. These recordings show REM sleep atonia with an awake EEG pattern.

HYPNIC JERKS

Hypnic jerks or "sleep starts" are physiologic phenomena without any pathologic significances that occur at sleep onset in many individuals with normal sleep functions. Episodes are associated with sudden, brief myoclonic jerks of the limbs or whole body that last for a few seconds. Sometimes, these jerks are accompanied by sensory phenomena, such as a sensation of falling; rarely have pure sensory "sleep starts" been described. Episodes may be triggered by stress, fatigue, or sleep deprivation. "Sleep starts" occur in up to 70% of the general population, and mainly involve the legs but sometimes affect the arms and head. Intensification of hypnic jerks may cause sleep-onset insomnia and occasionally may be mistaken for myoclonic seizures.

RHYTHMIC MOVEMENT DISORDER

Rhythmic movement disorder occurs mostly in infants younger than 18 months of age, is occasionally associated with mental retardation, and is rarely familial. It is a sleep–wake transition disorder with three characteristic movements: head banging, head rolling, and body rocking. Rhythmic movement disorder is a benign condition and the patient outgrows the episodes.

SLEEP TALKING

Sleep talking (somniloquy) is a benign phenomenon that consists of speech or sounds uttered by patients during sleep without awareness of behavior. Sleep talking becomes a problem when it occurs frequently and is loud enough to disturb the sleep of others. Reports of a dialogue occurring between two sleepers, neither of whom recall it on awakening, exists. Sleep talking most commonly occurs in NREM stages I and II and REM sleep; rarely, it occurs in SWS.

NOCTURNAL LEG CRAMPS

Nocturnal leg cramps are intensely painful sensations that are accompanied by muscle tightness occurring during sleep. These spasms usually last for a few seconds but sometimes persist for several minutes. Cramps during sleep are generally associated with awakening. Many normal individuals experience nocturnal leg cramps. Causes remain unknown. Local massage or movement of the limbs usually relieves the cramps.

BRUXISM

Bruxism (tooth grinding) occurs most commonly in individuals between ages 10 and 20 years and is also commonly noted in children with mental retardation or cerebral palsy. Bruxism is noted most prominently during NREM stages I and II and REM sleep. Episodes are characterized by stereotypical tooth grinding and are often precipitated by anxiety, stress, and dental disease. Occasionally, familial cases have been described.

BENIGN NEONATAL SLEEP MYOCLONUS

Benign neonatal sleep myoclonus occurs during the first few weeks of life and is generally seen in NREM sleep but sometimes during REM sleep. Episodes often occur in clusters and involve arms, legs, and (sometimes) trunk. Movements consist of jerky flexion, extension, abduction, and adduction. The condition is benign and requires no treatment.

ASSESSMENT AND TREATMENT OF PARASOMNIAS

Approaches to patients with parasomnias should follow the guidelines described in Chapter 7. PSG study is not routinely indicated in uncomplicated and typical parasomnias. PSG is, however, indicated in patients who experience unusual or atypical parasomnias or whose behaviors are violent or otherwise potentially injurious to themselves or others. Video-PSG recording should be performed to correlate behavior with PSG recordings.

Most of these parasomnias require no special treatment. The majority of subjects who experience NREM motor parasomnias (i.e., partial arousal disorders) require no treatment except preventive measures. Subjects must be protected from injuring themselves or others, a goal that is accomplished by arranging furniture, using padded mattresses, and paying particular attention to doors and windows. In severe cases in which spells occur almost every night, or if the patient is a child who is away sleeping with others, small doses of benzodiazepines (clonazepam) or tricyclic antidepressants (e.g., imipramine) may be used for a short period.

Rhythmic movement disorder, benign neonatal sleep myoclonus, and hypnic jerks are conditions that require no treatment. In cases of intensified hypnic jerks causing insomnia, patients should be reassured and the intensity of episodes may be reduced by treatment with clonazepam or zolpidem at bedtime.

Bruxism generally does not require any specific treatment unless it becomes chronic, causing symptoms such as wearing down of the teeth, headache, or facial pain. A tooth guard may be used to prevent tooth damage and muscle relaxants at bedtime may also be used.

Most cases of RBD respond dramatically to small doses of clonazepam (e.g., 0.5–2.0 mg at night).

19

Sleep Disorders in the Elderly

It is important to realize that no standard definition of the term *elderly* exists. For the sake of discussion in this chapter, elderly persons are defined as those individuals who are aged 65 years and older. In 1900, 4% of the American population was older than 65 years of age, a figure that will increase to 13% in 2000 and is estimated to reach 21% by 2050. Elderly individuals are at risk for sleep disturbances owing to a variety of factors, including social and psychosocial problems; increasing prevalence of concurrent medical, psychiatric, and neurologic illnesses; increasing use of medications and alcohol; and changes in body physiology and circadian rhythms.

CHANGES IN ELECTROENCEPHALOGRAPHY, SLEEP ARCHITECTURE, AND CIRCADIAN RHYTHMS IN OLD AGE

In elderly patients, a progressive slowing of alpha frequency intermixed with an increase in fast activity occurs in awake electroencephalography (EEG). Alpha-blocking and photic driving responses to intermittent photic stimulation are also diminished. These findings may be related to the nonspecific structural changes that occur in the central nervous system (e.g., loss of neurons in various locations, loss of dendritic spines, and lipofuscin accumulation). Whether these EEG changes are correlated with cerebral blood flow remains controversial. Other EEG changes occurring in old age include the presence of focal slow waves in the temporal region (particularly the left temporal region, often called *benign temporal delta transients of the elderly*) occasionally associated with sharp transients. Transient bursts of anteriorly dominant rhythmic delta waves may also occur during the early stage of sleep in elderly subjects.

In addition to awake EEG changes, other changes during sleep occur in the elderly. Sleep fragmentation due to frequent awakenings and sleep stage shifts occurs. Nighttime sleep may be decreased, but

Table 19.1
Changes in electroencephalography (EEG) and sleep architecture in old age

---

Awake EEG
   Progressive slowing of alpha frequency in the EEG
   Occasional focal transient slow and sharp waves in temporal regions
Sleep architecture
   Frequent awakenings with stage shifts and sleep fragmentation
   Early morning awakening
   Reduction of slow wave sleep
   Reduction of EEG delta amplitudes
   Increased stage I nonrapid eye movement sleep
   Decreased total nocturnal sleep
   Reduced total rapid eye movement sleep time but normal rapid eye
      movement percentage

---

because elderly individuals often take daytime naps, their 24-hour total sleep times are no different from those of young adults. Sleep changes that occur with advancing age may be summarized as follows: frequent stage shifts; reduction of slow wave sleep (SWS) (nonrapid eye movement stages III and IV) and EEG amplitude of delta waves; increased stage I caused by frequent arousals; decreased total nocturnal sleep; and a reduction of total rapid eye movement (REM) sleep time (with a normal REM percentage in relation to total sleep time).

Table 19.1 lists the physiologic changes that occur in EEG and sleep architecture in old age.

Circadian rhythm changes in the elderly result from fundamental changes in social (including family) interaction, as well as intrinsic changes in circadian rhythm related to pathologic alterations in the suprachiasmatic nuclei. The strong monophasic circadian rhythm of youth gives way to polyphasic ultradian rhythm in old age. Frequent awakenings occurring at night with reduction of wakefulness are accompanied by increased daytime naps. Phase advance also occurs in the elderly—that is, a tendency to go to sleep and awaken early exists. These changes may result from age-related changes in core body temperature rhythm. In elderly individuals, the amplitude of temperature rhythm is attenuated and phase is advanced.

PHYSIOLOGIC CHANGES IN THE ELDERLY

Striking changes occur in autonomic nervous system functions in elders. The most consistent abnormalities are increased muscle sympathetic nerve activity and elevated plasma concentration of the sympathetic neurotransmitter norepinephrine.

Thermoregulation is impaired in old age, making elderly individuals susceptible to hypothermia and hyperthermia.

Orthostatic hypotension commonly occurs in elderly patients and may be owing to impaired baroreflex responsiveness and neuroeffector function. A clear-cut decline in regional cerebral blood flow, noted more in gray than white matter, occurs in advancing age. This decline in cerebral blood flow appears to be related to a progressive decrease in cerebral metabolic rate and, possibly, morphologic changes in neurons in the brains of elderly individuals. The decrease of cerebral blood flow that occurs during SWS and the increase that occurs during REM sleep are similar in subjects of all ages with normal sleep functions. In elderly patients with sleep apnea, however, this decrease during SWS becomes excessive, placing elderly individuals at increasing risks for sudden death and development of stroke when combined with hypoxemia related to sleep apnea.

Age-related changes in the respiratory system and pulmonary function include reductions of vital capacity, chest wall compliance, diffusion capacity, elastic recoil, and arterial oxygen tension; a mismatched ventilation-perfusion ratio; decreased respiratory muscle strength; and respiratory center sensitivity. A higher incidence of periodic breathing at night, including Cheyne-Stokes breathing and snoring, exists in elderly patients.

Penile erection occurs during REM sleep. This REM-related penile tumescence shows a linear decrease from youth to old age.

The most striking change occurring in the endocrine system is a diminution of sleep-related growth hormone release. Whether this decreased release is related to a reduction of SWS is not known. In subjects older than 50 years of age, progressive changes in thyroid function also occur, causing modest decreases in serum triiodothyronine concentration and minimal changes in thyroid-stimulating hormone and thyroxin concentrations. Finally, serum melatonin concentration shows an age-related decrease in old age. Impaired melatonin secretion has been reported to be associated with sleep complaints in the elderly. Table 19.2 lists the physiologic changes that occur in different body systems in the elderly.

SLEEP COMPLAINTS IN OLD AGE

Persistent insomnia is an important late life complaint. A high incidence of depression with insomnia occurs in elderly patients. In one study, the prevalence of insomnia was 12% and the incidence was

Table 19.2
Physiologic changes in different body systems in the elderly

Autonomic nervous system changes
  Increased muscle sympathetic nerve activity
  Elevated plasma norepinephrine
  Orthostatic hypotension related to impaired baroreflex responsiveness
Cardiovascular changes
  Decline in regional cerebral blood flow caused by progressive decrease in
    cerebral metabolic rate
Respiratory system
  Reduced vital capacity, respiratory muscle strength, chest wall compliance,
    diffusion capacity, elastic recoil, arterial oxygen tension, and respira-
    tory center sensitivity
  Increased incidence of periodic breathing, including Cheyne-Stokes res-
    piration
Endocrine changes
  Diminution of sleep-related growth hormone release
  Progressive decrease in thyroid function
  Age-related decrease in serum melatonin concentration
Thermoregulation: impaired in old age
Nocturnal penile tumescence: rapid eye movement–related penile tumescence
  shows a linear decrease

7.3%. For hypersomnia, the figures for prevalence and incidence were 1.6% and 1.8%, respectively. It is also noted that persistent and debilitating complaints of insomnia occur in late-life spousal bereavement. In another study, an overall prevalence of 35% for insomnia complaints (more in women) existed among 1,017 noninstitutionalized elderly individuals. Insomnia complaints are more prevalent among women, whites, and individuals who experience depression, pain, and poor health.

Foley et al., in the National Institute on Aging's multicentered, epidemiologic study, conducted interviews of more than 9,000 persons aged 65 years and older from three communities in the United States. Authors observed at least one of the following complaints in more than half of the subjects: trouble falling asleep, multiple awakenings, early morning awakening, daytime naps, and tiredness. These complaints occurred more commonly in women than in men and were often associated with respiratory symptoms, depression, nonprescription and prescription medication, poor self-esteem, and physical disabilities. The authors also noted that 33% of men and 19% of women reported snoring, and 13% of men and 4% of women experienced apneas. Excessive daytime somnolence (EDS) is often associated with a fragmentation of nocturnal sleep that may be caused by the following factors: sleep-disordered breathing; periodic limb movements in sleep (PLMS); changes in circadian rhythms of temperature, alertness, and sleepiness; and social time cues.

In demented elderly subjects, nocturnal agitation, night wandering, shouting, and incontinence contribute to a variety of sleep disturbances. Many factors contribute to the pathogenesis of nocturnal agitation, including loss of social zeitgebers and circadian time keeping, sleep apnea, REM-related parasomnias, low ambient light, and cold sensitivity.

An important behavioral disturbance occurring during sleep late in life is snoring. According to Lugaresi and colleagues, approximately 65% of men and 40% of women between the ages of 41 and 64 years are habitual snorers.

The high frequency of sleep complaints in aged individuals may be related to the physiologic sleep changes of normal aging as well as to concomitant medical, psychiatric, neurologic, and other disorders prevalent in this group. Based on an extrapolation of survey data, it can be concluded that older individuals who sleep less than 5 hours or more than 9 hours a day may be at a greater risk for death.

COMMON SLEEP DISORDERS IN OLD AGE

Prevalence and intensity of sleep disturbances increase with age. Some common sleep disorders that have been recognized in elderly individuals include insomnia; sleep apnea syndrome; PLMS; sleep disturbances secondary to a variety of medical or psychiatric illnesses, particularly depression; sleep disturbances associated with dementia, particularly Alzheimer's type, and other neurodegenerative diseases (e.g., Parkinson's disease); sleep disturbances related to abuse of alcohol and sedative-hypnotic drugs; restless legs syndrome; parasomnias; and circadian rhythm sleep disorders (Table 19.3). Although narcolepsy is a disease with an onset occurring earlier than in old age, it is a life-line condition; therefore, it may be noted in elderly individuals.

Prevalences of sleep-related breathing disorders, PLMS, and snoring are greater among elderly patients. Prevalence of sleep apnea increases with age and is greater in men than in women (although it is greater in menopausal women than in premenopausal women). In various studies, prevalence rates for sleep apnea—defined as repetitive episodes of upper airway obstruction—in elderly patients have been estimated to range from 5.6% to 70.0%. A lack of consistency in study methods—

Table 19.3
Common sleep disorders in old age

Sleep-related breathing disorders
Periodic limb movements in sleep
Restless legs syndrome
Medical disorders causing sleep dysfunction
Sleep disorders associated with psychiatric illnesses
Neurodegenerative disorders
Drug and alcohol abuse
Parasomnias—commonly rapid eye movement sleep behavior disorder
Circadian rhythm disorders, particularly advanced sleep phase syndrome

such as sampling different populations without using a random sampling method, small sample size, or using different criteria to define sleep apnea—exists (see Chapter 10). Another problem occurs in defining the apnea index (AI) and respiratory disturbance index (RDI) and in assessing the clinical significances of an AI or RDI of 5. It is, therefore, difficult to generalize about the prevalence of sleep apnea in elderly people from these studies.

The relationship that exists between sleep apnea or sleep-disordered breathing and increased morbidity or mortality also remains controversial. Some surveys find that severe sleep-disordered breathing (e.g., breathing with an RDI of 30 or greater) is associated with significantly shorter patient survival rates, but that the RDI itself is not an independent predictor of death. Other confounding variables such as age, hypertension, and cardiovascular or pulmonary disease may be responsible for increased morbidity or mortality. Chronologic age may be the single most important determinant of increased morbidity and mortality in sleep-disordered breathing.

Insomnia and EDS are the two most common symptoms occurring in elderly individuals. A high incidence of insomnia exists in elderly patients, particularly in elderly women (see Chapter 11). A high prevalence of snoring occurring in elderly individuals may be the forerunner of full-blown sleep apnea syndrome. In diagnosing sleep apnea syndrome, questioning patients' bed partners is important. A patient history of loud snoring, with periods of cessation of breathing at night accompanied by EDS and daytime fatigue, suggests sleep apnea syndrome (see Chapter 10).

PLMS is reported more often in older normal subjects than in younger ones. PLMS may be related to sleep–wake disruption and disturbances of circadian sleep–wake rhythms in elderly individuals. Twenty-five percent to 35% of subjects ages 65 years and older may experience PLMS. Many investigators think that PLMS associated with arousals may cause insomnia, but this assumption remains somewhat controversial. Restless legs syndrome (RLS) is associated with PLMS in 80% of these cases. RLS is primarily a lifelong condition; its prevalence increases with age and symptoms may occur initially in old age. Further details of RLS have been described in Chapter 13.

A variety of general medical disorders and psychiatric illnesses may be associated with sleep disturbances (see Chapters 14 and 15). Important causes of sleep disturbances in the elderly are Alzheimer's disease and related dementia, as well as Parkinson's disease. Nocturnal confusional episodes (or sundowning syndrome) requiring antipsychotic medications have been described as existing in many demented elderly individuals (see Chapter 14).

A careful drug and alcohol history is important in assessing elderly individuals because they often take a variety of medications, including sedative-hypnotics for associated medical conditions and over-the-counter drugs to promote sleep. Sleeping medications produce secondary drug-related insomnia. Alcohol worsens sleep disturbances and may exacerbate existing sleep apnea syndrome.

An important parasomnia occurring in the elderly is rapid eye movement sleep behavior disorder (RBD). Sometimes, sleepwalking and night terrors have been described as occurring in elderly individuals, although these are generally present in children or adolescents. If, however, a relatively sudden onset of sleepwalking or night terrors occurs in an elderly person, the existence of an acute neurologic condition should be suspected and excluded by appropriate laboratory investigations. RBD can be confirmed by a patient's bed partner and by simultaneous video-polysomnographic (PSG) evaluation at night (see Chapter 18).

Frequent awakenings occurring during the night and early morning are noted commonly in elderly individuals. Sleep characteristics show an advanced phase that is also noted in other circadian rhythms such as body temperature and cortisol rhythms and timing of REM sleep. It has been suggested that circadian rhythm disorders may be caused by changes occurring in the circadian pacemaker with advancing age (e.g., a reduction of the number of neurons in the suprachiasmatic nucleus, the central pacemaker). Appropriately timed exposures to bright light might change circadian phase; thus, bright light therapy may be able to correct circadian sleep disorders in older individuals. Further research is needed in this area, however.

ASSESSMENT OF SLEEP DISORDERS
IN THE ELDERLY

Diagnostic evaluation should begin with a careful clinical assessment followed by appropriate laboratory investigations. Clinical assessment should consist of sleep, medical, drug, and psychiatric histories. A general approach for making clinical assessments is described in Chapter 7; only points relevant for assessing elders are emphasized in this section. An important point to remember in taking patient histories is that the sleep in elderly individuals becomes polyphasic, associated with frequent daytime naps and less sleep at night. Therefore, every daytime nap is not necessarily indicative of EDS. It is important, therefore, to obtain a patient's complete 24-hour sleep–wakefulness pattern. Elderly subjects must understand the significance of daytime fatigue, which may result either from insomnia at night or EDS.

Inquiries should be made regarding family history of sleep disorders. Certain sleep disorders (e.g., narcolepsy, hypersomnia, sleep apnea, sleep walking, night terrors, and restless legs syndrome) may have family histories. It is important to keep a sleep diary or log and to question the patient's bed partner or other caregivers about sleep disturbances. Keeping a sleep diary may help assess the 24-hour sleep–wake pattern. The bed partner or caregiver should be questioned carefully because he or she may have clues to aid in a diagnosis of sleep apnea syndrome. For example, excessive loud snoring, temporary cessation of breathing, or restless movements in bed are often indicative of sleep apnea syndrome or PLMS.

It is important to obtain an elderly patient's complete medical history because older individuals often experience a variety of medical disorders, including congestive cardiac failure, hypertension, ischemic heart disease, chronic bronchopulmonary disorders, gastrointestinal disorders, arthritis or musculoskeletal pain syndrome, cancer, chronic renal disorders, endocrinopathies, and a variety of neurologic disorders. All of these conditions may disrupt sleep by virtue of uncomfortable symptoms or due to the medications prescribed for them. Therefore, elderly patients often complain of insomnia, but sometimes they complain of hypersomnia as well.

It is important to obtain a patient's drug history because many medications can cause insomnia (see Chapter 11).

Psychophysiologic and psychiatric problems are common causes of insomnia in elderly patients. Elderly individuals with insomnia can have a variety of psychological and psychiatric problems such as anxiety, depression, organic psychosis, and obsessive-compulsive neurosis. A patient who experiences depression complains of early morning awakenings, whereas a patient with obsessive-compulsive neurosis experiences difficulty initiating sleep. Some drugs may increase nightmares. Marital and sexual problems may give rise to interpersonal problems that cause sleep disturbances, particularly insomnia.

Most sleep disturbances in elders can be diagnosed by careful history and physical examination. For some conditions, however, laboratory assessment is important. Two important laboratory tests are PSG study and Multiple Sleep Latency Test (MSLT). In sleep apnea syndrome, all-night PSG study is important in quantifying and determining the severity of sleep-related respiratory disturbance. This condition is treatable, so it is important to make a correct diagnosis. MSLT and PSG studies are also important for diagnosing narcolepsy, although in elderly people this diagnosis may have been made many years earlier. All-night video recordings are necessary to diagnose some conditions such as RBD or nocturnal seizures. Appropriate tests should be performed if other medical and neurologic disorders are suspected.

TREATMENT OF SLEEP DISORDERS IN THE ELDERLY

The objective of treatment is to improve quality of life and reduce risks of mortality and morbidity. Table 19.4 lists various treatment considerations for sleep disturbances in the elderly.

Indications for Treatment of Obstructive Sleep Apnea Syndrome

These treatments have been described in Chapter 10.

Table 19.4
Treatment considerations for sleep disturbances in the elderly

---

General measures
Treat obstructive sleep apnea syndrome
Treat insomnia using both nonpharmacologic and pharmacologic measures
Pharmacologic treatment of restless legs syndrome and periodic limb
    movements in sleep
Appropriate measures for circadian rhythm disorders
Special pharmacologic considerations
Situational and lifestyle considerations
Measures for nocturnal confusional episodes
Exercise program

Indications for Treatment of Insomnia

Multiple factors are responsible for insomnia in elderly individuals, therefore, evaluation and treatment of insomnia should be multidisciplinary. The first step in treatment is the elimination or avoidance of factors causing insomnia. The next important general measure is paying attention to sleep hygiene. For more information on the treatment of insomnia, see Chapter 11.

PLMS is a condition occurring in elderly patients, but its incidence and natural history are unknown. Even the relationship that exists between PLMS and insomnia is not clear. Therefore, any pharmacologic treatment for PLMS is subject to controversy and the long-term effect of treatment on patients is unknown. For selective cases in which PLMS clearly disrupts sleep, therapy may be indicated (see Chapter 13).

Circadian rhythm disorder, another important cause of insomnia, results from changes in the daily routine or sleep pattern, shift work, or transmedian travel. Therefore, environmental control and adequate counseling should be the first lines of treatment.

When a medical or psychiatric disorder causes insomnia, appropriate treatment should be directed toward the primary condition. In the case of depression in the elderly, appropriate treatment with a sedative antidepressant (e.g., amitriptyline, doxepin, or trazodone) may be instituted.

Medical conditions, such as cardiac failure, hypo- or hyperthyroidism, respiratory disorders, arthritis and other painful conditions, and gastroesophageal reflux disease, should be treated appropriately. Medications (e.g., theophylline or steroids) may cause sleep disturbance.

For transient or temporary sleep disturbances, short-term intermittent use of hypnotics and sedative tricyclics may be used. Long-term use of hypnotics is not recommended. The drug of choice for insomnia in the elderly is a benzodiazepine or zolpidem (see Chapter 11). Melatonin has received considerable attention as a hypnotic, based mostly on anecdotal rather than scientific evidence. Melatonin replacement therapy, however, may be beneficial in a subgroup of elderly insomniac patients with melatonin deficiency.

SPECIAL PHARMACOLOGIC CONSIDERATIONS IN THE ELDERLY

Drug metabolism and pharmacokinetics show changes in the elderly, and therefore it is important to start with a dose smaller than that required by younger subjects and gradually increase it depending on the response. It is also important to obtain a drug history to prevent drug interactions and exacerbation of sleep disturbances by hypnotics and other agents.

SITUATIONAL AND LIFESTYLE CONSIDERATIONS

Lifestyle factors are different for elderly patients. Retirement disturbs sleep–wake schedules; a so-called empty nest syndrome develops when children leave home; and bereavement over the death of a spouse or close friend may lead to loneliness and depression with attendant sleep disturbance. Other causes of sleep disorders in the elderly include institutionalization, prolonged bed rest, poor sleep hygiene, unsatisfactory bed environment, poor dietary habits, and caffeine and alcohol consumption.

TREATMENT OF SLEEP CYCLE CHANGES RELATED TO AGE

Treatment consists of educating patients about sleep disruption in old age, discouraging multiple naps, and urging participation in special interests, activities, and hobbies. The role of appropriately timed exposure to bright light in treating sleep maintenance insomnia and other circadian rhythm sleep disorders in elderly individuals remains to be determined.

TREATMENT OF SITUATIONAL STRESS

Patients should be given supportive psychotherapy and behavioral modification treatments as well as clear explanations of methods for reducing stress and sleeplessness.

TREATMENT OF NOCTURNAL CONFUSIONAL EPISODES

Treatment of nocturnal confusional episodes should be directed toward precipitating or causal factors. Often, episodes are precipitated when patients are transferred from their homes to institutions. As much as possible, the home environment should be preserved. Darkness of night often precipitates episodes, so a night-light is helpful. A careful drug history should be obtained and medications that are not absolutely necessary should be gradually reduced and eliminated. The treatment of choice for nocturnal confusion episodes is high-potency antipsychotics such as haloperidol and thiothixene.

TREATMENT OF MEDICATION-INDUCED SLEEP–WAKEFULNESS DISTURBANCES

Some medications cause insomnia, whereas others cause EDS. Patients should gradually eliminate drugs that are not essential and avoid alcohol, caffeine, and smoking.

EXERCISE PROGRAM

Exercise, particularly 5–6 hours before sleep, is thought to have a beneficial effect on sleep quality. In one study, a regular, moderate intensity, endurance exercise program showed improvements in sleep quality in older adults with moderate sleep complaints.

20

Pediatric Sleep Disorders

Despite a high prevalence of sleep disturbance in a large number of children, pediatric sleep disorders remain a neglected field. Several surveys confirm that approximately 25% of children aged 1–5 years are expected to experience some form of sleep problems. Mentally handicapped children and those with attention-deficit hyperactivity disorder experience higher rates of sleep disorders than do children without disorders. It should be remembered that normal sleep in newborns, infants, and children is different from that in adults (see Chapter 1). By age 6 months, a full-term normal infant should sleep through the night. However, if bedtime problems or nighttime awakenings continue to occur after that age, causes should be identified and corrected. Children experience the same sleep disorders as do adults, but presentations are somewhat different in children than in adults. Some problems are common among the pediatric population and some are distinctive. Some common sleep problems in children (Table 20.1) include a variety of parasomnias such as confusional arousals, sleep walking, sleep terrors, sleep talking, nightmares, sleep enuresis, bruxism, and rhythmic movement disorder; sleeplessness owing to specific childhood onset disorder or food allergy; excessive daytime somnolence (EDS) (e.g., narcolepsy or obstructive sleep apnea); and delayed or advanced sleep phase syndrome. Adjustment sleep disorder, limit setting sleep disorder, sleep onset association disorder, nocturnal eating (drinking) syndrome, and colic are some distinct sleep disorders causing insomnia in infants and children.

SPECIFIC SLEEP DISORDERS IN CHILDREN

Classifications of sleep disorders in children are similar to those in adults and follow classifications suggested by the International Classification of Sleep Disorders (ICSD). Extrinsic sleep disorders, however, are more common than intrinsic disorders in children. Presentations also differ

Table 20.1
Common sleep disorders in infants and children

Parasomnias
Adjustment sleep disorder
Sleep-onset association disorder
Limit-setting sleep disorder
Nocturnal eating (drinking) syndrome
Food allergy insomnia
Obstructive sleep apnea syndrome
Narcolepsy
Circadian rhythm sleep disorders

---

from children to adults. For example, obstructive sleep apnea syndrome symptoms in children are different than in adults (see section Obstructive Sleep Apnea Syndrome). Narcolepsy in children may present with prolonged periods of sleep rather than the short sleep attacks that occur in adults. Parent–child interactions are important determinants in understanding sleeplessness in children. Evaluation of sleepless or sleepy children should follow the same steps as evaluation in adults (see Chapter 7) except that histories are usually obtained from parents or caregivers. Unlike in adults, the impact of a child's sleep problem on the family determines the severity of the problem. It is important in cases of pediatric sleep disorders to obtain complete social histories, including family makeup, any occurrences of marital discord, alcohol, or drug abuse in parents, and other factors that may lead to stress in the home.

Adjustment Sleep Disorder

The ICSD defines *adjustment sleep disorder* as a type of sleep disturbance that is temporarily related to acute stress, conflict, or environmental changes that cause emotional arousal. Disturbance in most cases is brief. Either sleep-onset or maintenance insomnia or daytime sleepiness may be the presenting complaint. However, in children, insomnia is more common than sleepiness. If the external factor of stress is removed, the disorder resolves. If the disorder continues, however, an intrinsic sleep disorder, such as psychophysiologic insomnia, may be considered.

Sleep-Onset Association Disorder

Sleep-onset association disorder is a childhood sleep disorder characterized by an impairment of sleep onset due to the absence of a certain object or set of circumstances (e.g., bottle, pacifier, being rocked, watching television, or listening to the radio). Sleep is completely normal when the particular association is present. Treatment consists of training the child to make the transition from wake to sleep without expecting the parent's participation. It is best to start training children at approximately 6 months of age (the age when children are expected to sleep through the night). Parents must be consistent and persistent. The parents must be given sufficient support during the relearning process. During management, keeping a sleep diary and follow-up visits are important.

Limit-Setting Sleep Disorder

Limit-setting sleep disorder is exclusively a childhood sleep disorder characterized by stalling or refusing to go to sleep at an appropriate time as a result of inadequate enforcement of bedtime by the caretaker. When limit-setting is imposed, sleep onset is normal. The condition usually resolves as the child grows.

Nocturnal Eating (Drinking) Syndrome

The ICSD defines *nocturnal eating (drinking) syndrome* as a condition characterized by recurrent awakenings with an inability to return to sleep without eating or drinking. This condition is common during infancy and early childhood. Treatment involves gradual withdrawal from eating or drinking behavior.

Food Allergy Insomnia

Food allergy insomnia is a condition in which young children become allergic to cow's milk protein with severe sleep disruption. Symptoms begin whenever cow's milk is introduced into the diet and consist of sleep onset and maintenance difficulty with frequent awakenings. Systemic signs of milk allergy may be minimal or absent. Symptoms resolve within days to weeks on switching to a hypoallergenic formula. Regardless of treatment, however, spontaneous resolution occurs by age 2–4 years.

Obstructive Sleep Apnea Syndrome

Obstructive sleep apnea syndrome (OSAS) has been described as occurring in many children; however, certain differences exist between OSAS in children and OSAS in adults. Children may present with EDS, but common symptoms include hyperactivity and behavioral problems dur-

Table 20.2
Features of obstructive sleep apnea syndrome in children

Excessive daytime somnolence
Long history of nocturnal snoring
Disturbed sleep with frequent arousals
Hyperactivity and behavioral problems during the daytime
Impaired school performance
Intellectual changes
Sleep enuresis
Nocturnal diaphoresis
Delay in language development
Enlarged tonsils and adenoids
Systemic hypertension
Congestive cardiac failure

---

ing the daytime, impaired school performance, intellectual changes, increase in motor activity, disturbed sleep at night, and nocturnal snoring occurring for many months or years (Table 20.2). An important cause of OSAS in children is the enlargement of tonsils and adenoids. If OSAS is suspected, an overnight polysomnographic (PSG) study is indicated for documenting obstructive sleep apnea. In contrast to treatment in adults, removal of the tonsils and adenoids in children promotes symptomatic improvement. Some cases of sudden infant death syndrome (SIDS) are thought to be related to OSAS, but the relationship between SIDS and OSAS remains unproved and controversial. The most important factor in SIDS is sleeping in the prone position; therefore, every attempt must be made to keep the infant in the supine position.

Sleep Disorders Associated with Neurologic, General Medical, and Psychiatric Disorders

Neurologic disorders causing sleep disturbance in children include developmental and congenital abnormalities, mental retardation, chromosomal abnormalities, head injuries, brain tumor, metabolic and storage encephalopathies, and epilepsy (Table 20.3). Sleep complaints include insomnia, excessive sleepiness, and circadian rhythm sleep disorders. In all of these conditions, sleep abnormalities result from dysfunction of sleep–wake promoting neurons.

Management of such children is often difficult. Sometimes, pharmacologic intervention must be considered. Medications such as benzodiazepines, which are used to treat adult insomnia, are not as

Table 20.3
Common neurologic disorders causing sleep dysfunction in children

Developmental and congenital abnormalities
Mental retardation
Chromosomal abnormalities
Traumatic brain injuries
Brain tumors
Metabolic and storage encephalopathies
Epilepsy

effective in children. The best drug for treating insomnia in children is chloral hydrate, which must be given in sufficient doses to promote sleep. Doses as high as 50 mg/kg may be necessary in some patients. Other medications used include promethazine and clonidine. Clonidine is especially helpful in patients with attention-deficit hyperactivity disorder (ADHD). ADHD is probably a heterogeneous condition with soft neurologic signs. Characteristic sleep complaints in ADHD consist of restless sleep and awakenings at night. Stimulant medications with behavioral therapy are the mainstays of ADHD treatment.

Certain medical disorders that are particularly problematic in children include bronchial asthma with nighttime wheezing and awakenings, gastroesophageal reflux, chronic otitis media, and atopic dermatitis, which may be associated with poor sleep due to repeated awakenings at night (Table 20.4). In young infants, colic is the most common cause of sleep difficulty. Colic usually resolves by 3 months of age. The most successful treatment for postcolic sleep problems is the establishment and maintenance of a regular sleep schedule by parents.

Psychiatric disorders causing sleep disturbances in children are similar to those in adults. However, the most common psychiatric disorder affecting sleep in young children is anxiety. In cases of mild anxiety,

Table 20.4
Common medical disorders causing insomnia in children

Bronchial asthma with nighttime wheezing
Gastroesophageal reflux
Chronic otitis media
Atopic dermatitis
Infantile colic

reassurance is the only treatment necessary; in cases of long-standing and severe anxiety, however, family or individual counseling is needed.

Primary Enuresis

Primary enuresis is a condition of persistent bedwetting occurring in children older than 5 years of age that occurs in the absence of urologic, medical, psychiatric, or neurologic disorders. Enuretic episodes occur during all stages of sleep; however, they most commonly occur during the first third of the night. Treatment includes behavioral modification and conditioning techniques using enuresis alarms. If nonpharmacologic treatment is not successful, drug treatment with imipramine (25–75 mg, administered approximately one-half hour before sleep onset) may be used for approximately 6 months.

21

Sleep-Related Violence
and Forensic Issues

Sleep-related violent behavior is a symptom of many underlying disorders and not a disease by itself. Sleep-related violence, including homicide, suicide, and other types of aggression, has been reported. It is important to be knowledgeable about violent behaviors during sleep because of considerable personal, social, forensic, and legal implications. Complex behaviors without conscious awareness may arise out of nonrapid eye movement (NREM) or rapid eye movement (REM) sleep; these conditions are frequently treatable. Many abnormal and bizarre behaviors result from rapid oscillations of states (wakefulness, NREM, and REM sleep) or simultaneous occurrence of fragments of all three states. No evidence of significant psychopathology in the majority of these cases exists.

ETIOLOGIC FACTORS

Sleep-related violent behavior and acts are secondary to a variety of parasomnias and nonparasomnia disorders, including primary sleep disorders, neurologic, and psychogenic conditions (Table 21.1). A high incidence of violent aggressive behavior occurs in men, implying that testosterone is a factor in these complex behaviors. Violent or injurious behavior arises in absence of conscious awareness.

Clinical details of sleepwalking, sleep terror, and confusional arousals, which have given rise to many cases of sleep-related violence, have been described in Chapter 18. It is important to remember the triggering factors for these conditions for purposes of preventing incidences. Triggering factors include sleep deprivation, exhaustion, psychological stress, alcohol, and drugs. Patients are usually amnesic during these events, with only fragments of memory of these spells and no con-

Table 21.1
Etiologic factors for sleep-related violence

Primary sleep disorders
    Parasomnias
        Sleepwalking (SW)
        Sleep terrors (STs)
        Confusional arousals (CAs)
        Rapid eye movement (REM) sleep behavior disorder
        Intensified hypnic jerks
        Overlap parasomnias
            CAs/STs/SW
            Nonrapid eye movement/REM
    Nonparasomnia disorders
        Obstructive sleep apnea syndrome
        Narcolepsy with automatic behavior
        Idiopathic hypersomnia with sleep drunkenness
Neurologic causes
    Nocturnal seizures, including nocturnal paroxysmal dystonia, episodic
        nocturnal wanderings, and paroxysmal arousals
    Cerebral degenerative disorders causing nocturnal agitation and delirium
Psychiatric disorders
    Psychogenic dissociative states (waking and sleeping period)
    Malingering
    Munchausen syndrome
    Drug- and alcohol-related hypersomnia and sleep violence

---

scious wakefulness. Therefore, patients who experience these dysfunctions cannot be responsible for their acts.

Patients with obstructive sleep apnea syndrome (OSAS) experience frequent arousals that may sometimes trigger confusional arousals and sleep walking, causing abnormal motor manifestations and violent behavior.

Well-documented cases of somnambulistic homicide, attempted homicide, and suicide exist. Cases of murders and other crimes committed during states of sleep drunkenness and sleep apnea have been reported.

The neural basis of aggression and rage in these conditions remains undetermined. Environmental, social, and genetic factors may be contributing factors.

Rapid eye movement sleep behavior disorder (RBD) is a well-known REM parasomnia causing violent and injurious behavior both to the patient and his or her bed partners. The condition is reviewed in Chapter 18.

PSYCHOGENIC DISSOCIATIVE STATE

Psychogenic dissociative state is characterized by complex and often injurious behavior noted occasionally during apparent sleep periods at night. Polysomnographic (PSG) study, however, shows an electroencephalogram (EEG) wakeful pattern during the abnormal behavior. Patients invariably give a history of physical or sexual abuse as a child.

STATUS DISSOCIATUS

In addition to the psychogenic dissociative state, a condition known as *status dissociatus* exists, which is an organic disorder characterized by a complete breakdown of state boundaries and can be considered an extreme form of RBD. During attacks, patients experience complex motor and behavioral manifestations, causing injury to themselves or their bed partners. PSG study shows features of wakefulness, NREM, and REM sleep, making it impossible to score sleep. For example, a mixture of sleep spindles, REMs, alpha intrusions, and absences of REM muscle atonia may occur. The condition may be precipitated by prolonged withdrawal from alcohol abuse and has been noted occasionally in patients with narcolepsy and olivopontocerebellar atrophy or after open-heart surgery. Fatal familial insomnia, a rare prion disease, is almost invariably associated with features of status dissociatus.

MALINGERING AND MUNCHAUSEN SYNDROME

Malingering and Munchausen syndrome, although rare, must be considered in cases of apparent sleep-related violence. Munchausen syndrome is characterized by fake physical symptoms with repeated hospitalizations and visits to numerous physicians.

SLEEP SEIZURES

Sleep-related seizures may result in violent, injurious, or homicidal behavior. Seizures originating from the orbitofrontal or medial frontal regions may present with complex motor activities. Partial complex seizures of temporal origin may also present with complex behavior.

Violence and aggression may be ictal, preictal, or postictal. Patients with sleep seizures often respond satisfactorily to appropriate anticonvulsant therapy.

EVALUATION OF PATIENTS WITH SLEEP-RELATED VIOLENCE

Extensive neurologic, neuropsychological, and psychiatric assessment is essential in the treatment of patients who experience sleep-related violence. Particular attention must be paid to sleep and other histories, as outlined in Chapter 7. Patient histories should be obtained from parents or caregivers if patients are children. Complex behaviors arising during the early part of the night are most suggestive of arousal disorders, whereas those arising in the later part of the night suggest RBD. Nocturnal seizures can occur at any part of the night but are more frequently noted within 1–2 hours of sleep onset. In case of nocturnal sleep seizures, a history of tongue biting or urinary incontinence suggests seizures rather than parasomnias.

Laboratory tests in cases of sleep-related violence should include PSG recordings (particularly video-PSG), as well as split-screen telemetry. In cases of suspected seizures, EEG with full compliment of electrodes covering the parasagittal and temporal areas should be obtained. Ambulatory monitoring may also be recorded in some patients. In psychogenic cases, psychological tests, including the Minnesota Multiphasic Personality Inventory, should be undertaken.

PRINCIPLES OF MANAGEMENT OF PATIENTS WITH SLEEP-RELATED VIOLENCE

Sleep-related violence is not recurrent. Prevention by early diagnosis and treatment before violence occurs is the best measure. Triggering factors should be avoided in cases of suspected arousal disorder. Appropriate measures taken to avoid injuries to self and others should be undertaken. It is important to avoid physically restraining subjects during episodes of confusional arousal, sleep walking, or sleep terrors because restraint may further aggravate conditions. Most behaviors generally stop after a few minutes. It is important to treat the underlying parasomnias with appropriate medications. Finally, counseling the patient and his or her family is essential for his or her understanding that violent or injurious behavior may arise in the absence of conscious awareness.

Table 21.2
Guidelines to determine the role of a specific sleep disorder in violence

---

The sleep disorder should be diagnosed by history or overnight video-polysomnographic study

The episode usually lasts a few minutes

The behavior is usually abrupt, impulsive, immediate, and without apparent motivation or premeditation

The victim may be the stimulus for arousal and merely happened to be present

Perplexity, horror, and lack of awareness without any attempt to escape or cover up the action are the striking features on regaining consciousness

Amnesia (complete or partial) for the event is a characteristic phenomenon

In cases of arousal disorders (sleep walking, sleep terror, or confusional episodes), the violent act may occur on awakening or attempted awakening from sleep, usually during first third of sleep at night and may have been precipitated by triggering factors (e.g., alcohol, hypnotics, or sleep deprivation)

Source: Adapted from MW Mahowald, CH Schenck. Sleep-Related Violence and Forensic Medicine Issues. In S Chokroverty (ed), Sleep Disorders Medicine: Basic Science, Technical Considerations and Clinical Aspects (2nd ed). Boston: Butterworth–Heinemann, 1999;729–739.

FORENSIC IMPLICATIONS

Many cases of sleep-related violence exist that have been decided in court. Some subjects have been convicted whereas others are acquitted. These cases are controversial and decisions are rather difficult. Legal implications have been discussed and debated by medical and legal professionals. Guidelines have been proposed to determine the roles of specific sleep disorders in particular violent acts (Table 21.2). The American Academy of Neurology and the American Sleep Disorders Association (now known as the American Academy of Sleep Medicine) have developed specific guidelines for expert testimony. A need for impartial testimony (without advocating for the plaintiff or defense) exists. Whether sleepwalking and other parasomnias can be legally classified as an insane or a noninsane automatism is the crucial question. Finally, the important point is to avoid "junk science" in the courtroom.

Appendix

Glossary of Terms*

Actigraph　A biomedical instrument for the measurement of body movement.

Active sleep　A term used in the phylogenetic and ontogenetic literature for the stage of sleep that is considered to be equivalent to REM sleep (see *REM sleep*).

Alpha activity　An alpha EEG wave or sequence of waves with a frequency of 8–13 Hz.

Alpha-delta sleep　Sleep in which alpha activity occurs during slow wave sleep. Because alpha-delta sleep is rarely seen without alpha occurring in other sleep stages, the term *alpha sleep* is preferred.

Alpha intrusion (-infiltration, -insertion, -interruption)　A brief superimposition of EEG alpha activity on sleep activities during a stage of sleep.

Alpha rhythm　An EEG rhythm with a frequency of 8–13 Hz in human adults that is most prominent over the parieto-occipital cortex when the eyes are closed. The rhythm is blocked by eye opening or other arousing stimuli. It is indicative of the awake state in most normal individuals and is most consistent and predominant during relaxed wakefulness, particularly with reduction of visual input. The amplitude is variable but typically is below 50 µV in adults. The alpha rhythm of an individual usually slows by 0.5–1.5 Hz and becomes more diffuse during drowsiness. The frequency range also varies with age; it is slower in children and older age groups than in young to middle-age adults.

Alpha sleep　Sleep in which alpha activity occurs during most, if not all, sleep stages.

Apnea　Cessation of airflow at the nostrils and mouth lasting at least 10 seconds. There are three types of apnea: obstructive, central, and mixed. Obstructive apnea is secondary to upper airway obstruction; central apnea is associated with a cessation of all respiratory movements; mixed apnea has both central and obstructive components.

---

*Adapted with the permission of the American Sleep Disorders Association, Rochester, Minnesota.

Apnea–hypopnea index   The number of apneic episodes (obstructive, central, and mixed) plus hypopneas per hour of sleep as determined by all-night polysomnography. Synonymous with *respiratory disturbance index*.

Apnea index   The number of apneic episodes (obstructive, central, and mixed) per hour of sleep as determined with all-night polysomnography. Sometimes a separate obstructive apnea index or central apnea index is used.

Arise time   The clock time that an individual gets out of bed after the final awakening of the major sleep episode (distinguished from final wake-up).

Arousal   An abrupt change from a deeper stage of non-REM sleep to a lighter stage, or from REM sleep to wakefulness, with the possibility of awakening as the final outcome. Arousal may be accompanied by increased tonic electromyographic activity and heart rate as well as body movements.

Arousal disorder   A parasomnia disorder presumed to be due to an abnormal arousal mechanism. Forced arousal from sleep can induce episodes. The classic arousal disorders are sleepwalking, sleep terrors, and confusional arousals.

Awakening   The return to the polysomnographically defined awake state from any non-REM or REM sleep stage. It is characterized by alpha and beta EEG activity, a rise in tonic electromyography, voluntary REMs, and eye blinks. This definition of awakenings is valid only insofar as the polysomnogram is paralleled by a resumption of a reasonably alert state of awareness of the environment.

Axial system   A means of presenting different types of information in a systematic manner using several "axes" to ensure that important information is not overlooked in light of a single major diagnosis. The International Classification of Sleep Disorders uses a three-axis system: axes A, B, and C.

Axis A   The first level of the axial system devised by the International Classification of Sleep Disorders. Axis A includes the sleep disorder diagnoses, modifiers, and associated code numbers.

Axis B   The second level of the axial system devised by the International Classification of Sleep Disorders. Axis B includes the sleep-related procedures, procedure features, and associated code numbers.

Axis C   The third level of the axial system devised by the International Classification of Sleep Disorders. Axis C includes nonsleep diagnoses and associated code numbers.

Baseline   The typical or normal state of an individual or of an investigative variable before an experimental manipulation.

Bedtime   The clock time at which one attempts to fall asleep, as differentiated from the clock time when one gets into bed.

Beta activity   A beta EEG wave or sequence of waves with frequency greater than 13 Hz.

Beta rhythm   An EEG rhythm in the range of 13–35 Hz, when the predominant frequency, beta rhythm, is usually associated with alert wakefulness or vigilance and is accompanied by a high tonic EMG. The amplitude of beta rhythm is variable but usually is below 30 μV. This rhythm may be drug induced.

Brain wave   Use of this term is discouraged. The preferred term is *EEG wave.*

Cataplexy   A sudden decrement in muscle tone and loss of deep tendon reflexes leading to muscle weakness, paralysis, or postural collapse. Cataplexy usually is precipitated by an outburst of emotional expression, notably laughter, anger, or startle. One of the symptom tetrad of narcolepsy. During cataplexy, respiration and voluntary eye movements are not compromised.

Cheyne-Stokes respiration   A breathing pattern characterized by regular "crescendo-decrescendo" fluctuations in respiratory rate and tidal volume.

Chronobiology   The science of temporal, primarily rhythmic, processes in biology.

Circadian rhythm   An innate, daily fluctuation of physiologic or behavioral functions, including sleep–wake states generally tied to the 24-hour daily dark–light cycle. Sometimes occurs at a measurably different periodicity (e.g., 23 or 25 hours) when light–dark and other time cues are removed.

Circasemidian rhythm   A biological rhythm that has a period length of approximately half a day.

Conditional insomnia   Insomnia produced by the development, during an earlier experience of sleeplessness, of conditioned arousal. Causes of the conditioned stimulus can include the customary sleep environment or thoughts of disturbed sleep. A conditioned insomnia is one component of psychophysiologic insomnia.

Constant routine   A chronobiological test of the endogenous pacemaker that involves a 36-hour baseline monitoring period followed by a 40-hour waking episode of monitoring with the individual on a constant routine of food intake, position, activity, and light exposure.

Cycle   Characteristic of an event exhibiting rhythmic fluctuations. One cycle is defined as the activity from one maximum or minimum to the next.

Deep sleep   Common term for combined non-REM stage III and IV sleep. In some sleep literature, deep sleep is applied to REM sleep because of its high awakening threshold to nonsignificant stimuli (see *"Intermediary" sleep stage; Light sleep*).

Delayed sleep phase   A condition that occurs when the clock hour at which sleep normally occurs is moved ahead in time within a given 24-hour sleep–wake cycle. This results in a temporarily displaced—that is, delayed—occurrence of sleep within the 24-hour cycle. The same term denotes a circadian rhythm sleep disturbance called *delayed sleep phase syndrome*.

Delta activity   EEG activity with a frequency of less than 4 Hz (usually 0.1–3.5 Hz). In human sleep scoring, the minimum characteristics for scoring delta waves are conventionally 75 µV amplitude (peak-to-peak) and 0.5 seconds' duration (2 Hz) or less.

Delta sleep stage   The stage of sleep in which EEG delta waves are prevalent or predominant—sleep stages III and IV, respectively (see *Slow wave sleep*).

Diagnostic criteria   Specific criteria established in the International Classification of Sleep Disorders to aid in determining the unequivocal presence of a particular sleep disorder.

Diurnal   Pertaining to daytime.

Drowsiness   A stage of quiet wakefulness that typically occurs before sleep onset. If the eyes are closed, diffuse slowed alpha activity usually is present, which then gives way to early features of stage I sleep.

Duration criteria   Criteria (acute, subacute, chronic) established in the International Classification of Sleep Disorders for determining the duration of a particular disorder.

Dyssomnia   A primary disorder of initiating and maintaining sleep or of excessive sleepiness. The dyssomnias are disorders of sleep or wakefulness per se; not a parasomnia.

Early morning arousal (early AM arousal)   Premature morning awakening.

Electroencephalogram (EEG)   A recording of the electrical activity of the brain by means of electrodes placed on the surface of the head. With the electromyogram and electro-oculogram, the EEG is one of the three basic variables used to score sleep stages and waking. Sleep recording in humans uses surface electrodes to record potential differences between brain regions and a neutral reference point, or simply between brain regions. Either the C3 or C4 placement (central region, according to the International 10-20 System) is referentially (referred to an earlobe) recorded as the standard electrode derivation from which state scoring is done.

Electromyogram (EMG)   A recording of electrical activity from the muscular system; in sleep recording, same as muscle activity or potential. The chin EMG, along with EEG and electro-oculography, is one of the three basic variables used to score sleep stages and waking. Sleep recording in humans typically uses surface electrodes to measure activity from the submental muscles. These reflect maximally the changes in resting activity of axial body muscles. The submental muscle EMG is tonically inhibited during REM sleep.

Electro-oculogram (EOG)   A recording of voltage changes resulting from shifts in position of the ocular gloves, as each glove is a positive (anterior) and negative (posterior) dipole; along with the EEG and electromyogram, one of the three basic variables used to score sleep stages and waking. Sleep recording in humans uses surface electrodes placed near the eyes to record the movement (incidence, direction, and velocity) of the eyeballs. REMs in sleep form one part of the characteristics of the REM sleep state.

End-tidal carbon dioxide   Carbon dioxide value usually determined at the nares by an infrared carbon dioxide gas analyzer. The value reflects the alveolar or pulmonary arterial blood carbon dioxide level.

Entrainment   Synchronization of a biological rhythm by a forcing stimulus such as an environmental time cue (see *Zeitgeber*). During entrainment, the frequencies of the two cycles are the same or are integral multiples of each other.

Epoch   A measure of duration of the sleep recording, typically 20–30 seconds in duration, depending on the paper speed of the polysomnograph. An epoch corresponds to one page of the polysomnogram.

Excessive sleepiness (-somnolence, -hypersomnia, excessive daytime sleepiness)   A subjective report of difficulty in maintaining the alert awake state, usually accompanied by a rapid entrance into sleep when the person is sedentary. May be due to an excessively deep or prolonged major sleep episode. Can be quantitatively measured by use of subjectively defined rating scales of sleepiness, or physiologically measured by electrophysiologic tests such as the Multiple Sleep Latency Test (see *Multiple Sleep Latency Test*). Most commonly occurs during the daytime; however, excessive sleepiness may be present at night in a person whose major sleep episode occurs during the daytime, such as a shift worker.

Extrinsic sleep disorders   Disorders that originate, develop, or arise from causes outside of the body. The extrinsic sleep disorders are a subgroup of the dyssomnias.

Final awakening   The duration of wakefulness after the final wake-up time until the arise time (lights on).

Final wake-up   The clock time at which an individual awakens for the last time before the arise time.

First-night effect   The effect of the environment and polysomnographic recording apparatus on the quality of the subject's sleep during the first night of recording. Sleep is usually of reduced quality compared to what would be expected in the subject's usual sleeping environment without electrodes and other recording procedure stimuli. The subject usually is habituated to the laboratory by the time of the second night of recording.

Fragmentation (of sleep architecture)   The interruption of any stage of sleep owing to the appearance of another stage or wakefulness, leading to disrupted non-REM–REM sleep cycles; often used to refer to the interruption of REM sleep by movement arousals or stage II activity. Sleep fragmentation connotes repetitive interruptions of sleep by arousals and awakenings.

Free-running   A chronobiological term that refers to the natural endogenous period of a rhythm when *Zeitgebers* are removed. In humans, it most commonly is seen in the tendency to delay some circadian rhythms, such as the sleep–wake cycle, by approximately 1 hour every day, when a person has an impaired ability to entrain or is without time cues.

Hertz   A unit of frequency; preferred to the synonymous expression *cycles per second.*

Hypercapnia   Elevated level of carbon dioxide in blood.

Hypersomnia   Excessively deep or prolonged major sleep period. May be associated with difficulty in awakening. Hypersomnia is primarily a diagnostic term (e.g., idiopathic hypersomnia); *excessive sleepiness* is preferred to describe the symptom.

Hypnagogic   Descriptor for events that occur during the transition from wakefulness to sleep.

Hypnagogic imagery (-hallucinations)   Vivid sensory images occurring at sleep onset, but particularly vivid with sleep-onset REM periods. A feature of narcoleptic naps, when the onset occurs with REM sleep.

Hypnagogic startle   A "sleep start" or sudden body jerk (hypnic jerk), observed normally just at sleep onset and usually resulting, at least momentarily, in awakening.

Hypnopompic (hypnopomic)   Descriptor of an occurrence during the transition from sleep to wakefulness at the termination of a sleep episode.

Hypopnea   An episode of shallow breathing (airflow reduced by at least 50%) during sleep lasting 10 seconds or longer, usually associated with a fall in blood oxygen saturation.

International Classification of Sleep Disorders sleep code   A code number of the International Classification of the Sleep Disorders that refers to modifying information of a diagnosis, such as associated symptom, severity, or duration of a sleep disorder.

Insomnia   Difficulty initiating or maintaining sleep. A term that is employed ubiquitously to indicate any and all gradations and types of sleep loss.

"Intermediary" sleep stage   A term sometimes used for non-REM stage II sleep (see *Deep sleep*; *Light sleep*). Often used, especially in the French literature, for stages combining elements of stage II and REM sleep.

Into-bed time   The clock time at which a person gets into bed. The into-bed time is synonymous with bedtime for many people, but not for those who spend time in wakeful activities in bed, such as reading, before attempting to sleep.

Intrinsic sleep disorders   Disorders that originate, develop, or arise from causes within the body. The intrinsic sleep disorders are a subgroup of the dyssomnias.

K-alpha   A K complex followed by several seconds of alpha rhythm; a type of microarousal.

K complex   A sharp, negative EEG wave followed by a high-voltage slow wave. The complex duration is at least 0.5 second, and may be accompanied by a sleep spindle. K complexes occur spontaneously during non-REM sleep, and begin and define stage II sleep. They are thought to be evoked responses to internal stimuli. They can also be elicited during sleep by external (particularly auditory) stimuli.

Light-dark cycle   The periodic pattern of light (artificial or natural) alternating with darkness.

Light sleep   A common term for non-REM sleep stage I and sometimes stage II.

Maintenance of Wakefulness Test   A series of measurements of the interval from lights out to sleep onset that is used in the assessment of the ability to remain awake. Subjects are instructed to try to remain awake in a darkened room when in a semireclined position. Long latencies to sleep are indicative of the ability to remain awake. This test is most useful for assessing the effects of medication on the ability to remain awake.

Major sleep episode   The longest sleep episode that occurs on a daily basis. Typically the sleep episode dictated by the circadian rhythm of sleep and wakefulness; the conventional or habitual time for sleeping.

Microsleep   An episode that lasts up to 30 seconds, during which external stimuli are not perceived. The polysomnogram suddenly shifts from waking characteristics to sleep. Microsleeps are associated with excessive sleepiness and automatic behavior.

Minimal criteria   Criteria of the International Classification of Sleep Disorders derived from the diagnostic criteria that provide the minimum features necessary for making a particular sleep disorder diagnosis.

Montage   The particular arrangement by which a number of derivations are displayed simultaneously in a polysomnogram.

Movement arousal   A body movement associated with an EEG pattern of arousal or a full awakening; a sleep-scoring variable.

Movement time   The term used in sleep record scoring to denote when EEG and electro-oculography tracings are obscured for more than half the scoring epoch because of movement. It is scored only when the preceding and subsequent epochs are in sleep.

Multiple Sleep Latency Test   A series of measurements of the interval from lights out to sleep onset that is used in the assessment of excessive sleepiness. Subjects are allowed a fixed number of opportunities to fall asleep during their customary awake period. Excessive sleepiness is characterized by short latencies. Long latencies are helpful in distinguishing physical tiredness or fatigue from true sleepiness.

Muscle tone   A term sometimes used for resting muscle potential or resting muscle activity (see *Electromyogram*).

Myoclonus   Muscle contractions in the form of abrupt jerks or twitches generally lasting less than 100 msec. The term should not be applied to the periodic leg movements of sleep that characteristically have a duration of 0.5–5.0 seconds.

Nap   A short sleep episode that may be intentionally or unintentionally taken during the period of habitual wakefulness.

Nightmare   An unpleasant and frightening dream that usually occurs in REM sleep. Occasionally called a dream anxiety attack, it is not a sleep (night) terror. Nightmare in the past has been used to indicate both sleep terror and dream anxiety attacks.

Nocturnal confusion   Episodes of delirium and disorientation close to or during nighttime sleep; often seen in the elderly and indicative of organic central nervous system deterioration.

Nocturnal dyspnea   Respiratory distress that may be minimal during the day but becomes quite pronounced during sleep.

Nocturnal penile tumescence   The natural periodic cycle of penile erections that occur during sleep, typically associated with REM sleep. The preferred term is *sleep-related erections*.

Nocturnal sleep   The typical "nighttime" or major sleep episode related to the circadian rhythm of sleep and wakefulness; the conventional or habitual time for sleeping.

Non-REM sleep   See *Sleep stages*.

Non-REM–REM sleep cycle (sleep cycle)   A period during sleep composed of a non-REM sleep episode and the subsequent REM sleep episode; each non-REM–REM sleep couplet is equal to one cycle. Any non-REM sleep stage suffices as the non-REM sleep portion of a cycle. An adult sleep period of 6.5–8.5 hours generally consists of four to six cycles. The cycle duration increases from infancy to young adulthood.

Non-REM sleep intrusion   An interposition of non-REM sleep, or a component of non-REM sleep physiology (e.g., elevated EMG, K complex, sleep spindle, delta waves) in REM sleep; a portion of non-REM sleep not appearing in its usual sleep cycle position.

Non-REM sleep period   The non-REM sleep portion of non-REM–REM sleep cycle; such an episode consists primarily of sleep stages III and IV early in the night and of sleep stage II later (see *Sleep cycle*; *Sleep stages*).

Obesity-hypoventilation syndrome   A condition of obese individuals who hypoventilate during wakefulness. Because the term can apply to several different disorders, its use is discouraged.

Paradoxical sleep   Synonymous with *REM sleep*, which is the preferred term.

Parasomnia   Disorder of arousal, partial arousal, or sleep stage transition, not a dyssomnia. It represents an episodic disorder in sleep (such as sleepwalking) rather than a disorder of sleep or wakefulness per se. May be induced or exacerbated by sleep.

Paroxysm   Phenomenon of abrupt onset that rapidly attains maximum intensity and terminates suddenly; distinguished from background activity. Commonly refers to an epileptiform discharge on the EEG.

Paroxysmal nocturnal dyspnea   Respiratory distress and shortness of breath due to pulmonary edema, which appears suddenly and often awakens the sleeper.

Penile buckling pressure   The amount of force applied to the glans of the penis sufficient to produce at least a 30-degree bend in the shaft.

Penile rigidity   The firmness of the penis as measured by the penile buckling pressure. Normally, the fully erect penis has maximum rigidity.

Period   The interval between the recurrence of a defined phase or moment of a rhythmic or regularly recurring event—that is, the interval between one peak or trough and the next.

Periodic leg movement   Rapid partial dorsiflexion of the foot at the ankle, extension of the big toe, and partial flexion of the knee and hip that occurs during sleep. The movements occur with a periodicity of 20–60 seconds in a stereotyped pattern lasting 0.5–5.0 seconds and are a characteristic feature of periodic limb movements in sleep disorder.

Periodic limb movements in sleep   See *Periodic leg movement*.

Phase advance   The shift of an episode of sleep or wake to an earlier position in the 24-hour sleep–wake cycle. A sleep period of 11 PM to 7 AM shifted to 8 PM to 4 AM represents a 3-hour phase advance (see *Phase delay*).

Phase delay   A shift of an episode of sleep or wake to a later time of the 24-hour sleep–wake cycle. It is the exact opposite of *phase advance*. These terms differ from common concepts of change in clock time; to effect a phase delay, the clock is moved ahead or advanced. In contrast, to effect a phase advance, the clock moves backward (see *Phase advance*).

Phase transition   One of the two junctures of the major sleep and wake phases in the 24-hour sleep–wake cycle.

Phasic event (-activity)   Brain, muscle, or autonomic event of a brief and episodic nature occurring in sleep; characteristic of REM sleep, such as eye movements or muscle twitches. Usually the duration is milliseconds to 2 seconds.

Photoperiod   The period of light in a light-dark cycle.

Pickwickian   Descriptor for an obese person who snores, is sleepy, and has alveolar hypoventilation. The term has been applied to many different disorders and therefore its use is discouraged.

PLM-arousal index   The number of sleep-related periodic leg movements per hour of sleep that are associated with an EEG arousal (see *Periodic leg movement*).

PLM index   The number of periodic leg movements per hour of total sleep time as determined by all-night polysomnography. Sometimes expressed as the number of movements per hour of non-REM sleep because the movements are usually inhibited during REM sleep (see *Periodic leg movement*).

PLM percentage   The percentage of total sleep time occupied with recurrent episodes of periodic leg movements.

Polysomnogram   The continuous and simultaneous recording of multiple physiologic variables during sleep (i.e., EEG, electro-oculography, electromyography—the three basic stage-scoring parameters—electrocardiogram, respiratory airflow, respiratory movements, leg movements, and other electrophysiologic variables.

Polysomnograph   A biomedical instrument for the measurement of physiologic variables of sleep.

Polysomnographic (-recording, -monitoring, -registration, -tracings)   Describes a recording on paper, computer disc, or tape of a polysomnogram.

Premature morning awakening   Early termination of the sleep episode, with inability to return to sleep, sometimes after the last of several awakenings. It reflects interference at the end, rather than at the commencement, of the sleep episode. A characteristic sleep disturbance of some people with depression.

Proposed sleep disorder   A disorder in which insufficient information is available in the medical literature to confirm the unequivocal existence of the disorder. A category of the International Classification of Sleep Disorders.

Quiet sleep   A term used to describe non-REM sleep in infants and animals when specific non-REM sleep stages I–IV cannot be determined.

REM sleep   Rapid eye movement sleep (see *Sleep stages*).

Record   The end product of the polysomnographic recording process.

Recording   The process of obtaining a polysomnographic record. The term is also applied to the end product of the polysomnographic recording process.

REM density (-intensity)   A function that expresses the frequency of eye movements per unit time during sleep stage REM.

REM sleep episode   The REM sleep portion of a non-REM–REM sleep cycle. Early in the night it may be as short as a half minute, in later cycles longer than an hour (see *Sleep stage REM*).

REM sleep intrusion   A brief interval of REM sleep appearing out of its usual position in the non-REM–REM sleep cycle; an interposition of REM sleep in non-REM sleep; sometimes appearance of a single, dissociated component of REM sleep (e.g., eye movements, "drop out" of muscle tone) rather than all REM sleep parameters.

REM sleep latency   The interval from sleep onset to the first appearance of stage REM sleep in the sleep episode.

REM sleep onset   The designation for commencement of a REM sleep episode. Sometimes also used as a shorthand term for a sleep-onset REM sleep episode (see *Sleep onset; Sleep-onset REM period*).

REM sleep percent   The proportion of total sleep time constituted by REM stage of sleep.

REM sleep rebound (recovery)   Lengthening and increase in frequency and density of REM sleep episodes, which results in an increase in REM sleep percent above baseline. REM sleep rebound follows REM sleep deprivation once the depriving influence is removed.

Respiratory disturbance index   The number of apneas (obstructive, central, or mixed) plus hypopneas per hour of total sleep time as determined by all-night polysomnography. Synonymous with *apnea-hypopnea index*.

Restlessness   Referring to quality of sleep, persistent or recurrent body movements, arousals, and brief awakenings in the course of sleep.

Rhythm   An event occurring with approximately constant periodicity.

Sawtooth waves   A form of theta rhythm that occurs during REM sleep and is characterized by a notched waveform. Occurs in bursts lasting as long as 10 seconds.

Severity criteria   Criteria for establishing the severity of a particular sleep disorder according to three categories: mild, moderate, or severe.

Sleep architecture   The non-REM–REM sleep stage and cycle infrastructure of sleep understood from the vantage point of the quantitative relationship of these components to each other. Often plotted in the form of a histogram.

Sleep cycle   Synonymous with the non-REM–REM sleep cycle.

Sleep efficiency (sleep efficiency index)   The proportion of sleep in the episode potentially filled by sleep (i.e., the ratio of total sleep time to time in bed).

Sleep episode   An interval of sleep that may be voluntary or involuntary. In the sleep laboratory, the sleep episode occurs from the time of lights out to the time of lights on. The major sleep episode is usually the longest one.

Sleep hygiene   Conditions and practices that promote continuous and effective sleep. These include regularity of bedtime and arise time; conformity of time spent in bed to the time necessary for sustained and individually adequate sleep (i.e., the total sleep time sufficient to avoid sleepiness when awake); restriction of alcohol and caffeine before bedtime; and using exercise, nutrition, and environmental factors as strategies to enhance, rather than disturb, restful sleep.

Sleepiness (somnolence, drowsiness)   Difficulty maintaining alert wakefulness so that a person falls asleep if not actively aroused. This is not simply a feeling of physical tiredness or listlessness. When sleepiness occurs in inappropriate circumstances, it is considered excessive sleepiness.

Sleep interruption   Breaks in sleep resulting in arousal and wakefulness (see *Fragmentation; Restlessness*).

Sleep latency   The duration of time from lights out to the onset of sleep.

Sleep log (-diary)   A daily, written record of a person's sleep–wake pattern, containing information such as time of retiring and arising, time in bed, estimated total sleep time, number and duration of sleep interruptions, quality of sleep, daytime naps, use of medication or consumption of caffeine, nature of waking activities.

Sleep-maintenance disorder (insomnia)   Difficulty maintaining sleep, once achieved; persistently interrupted sleep without difficulty falling asleep. Synonymous with *sleep continuity disturbance*.

Sleep mentation   The imagery and thinking experienced during sleep. Sleep mentation usually consists of combinations of images and thoughts during REM sleep. Imagery is vividly expressed in dreams involving all the senses in approximate proportion to their waking representations. Mentation is experienced generally less distinctly in non-REM sleep, but it may be quite vivid in stage II sleep, especially toward the end of the sleep episode. Mentation at sleep onset (hypnagogic reverie) can be as vivid as in REM sleep.

Sleep onset   The transition from waking to sleep, normally into non-REM stage I sleep but in certain conditions such as infancy and narcolepsy into stage REM sleep. Most polysomnographers accept EEG slowing; reduction and eventual disappearance of alpha activity; presence of EEG vertex sharp transients; and slow, rolling eye movements (the components of non-REM stage I) as sufficient criteria for sleep onset; others require appearance of stage II patterns (see *Sleep latency*; *Sleep stages*).

Sleep-onset REM period   The beginning of sleep by entrance directly into stage REM sleep. The onset of REM occurs within 10 minutes of sleep onset.

Sleep paralysis   Immobility of the body that occurs in the transition from sleep to wakefulness; a partial manifestation of REM sleep.

Sleep pattern (24-hour sleep–wake pattern)   A person's clock-hour schedule of bedtime and arise time as well as nap behavior; may include time and duration of sleep interruptions (see *Sleep–wake cycle*; *Circadian rhythm*; *Sleep log*).

Sleep-related erections   The natural periodic cycle of penile erections that occur during sleep, typically associated with REM sleep. Sleep-related erectile activity can be characterized as four phases: T-up (ascending tumescence), T-max (plateau maximal tumescence), T-down (detumescence), and T-zero (no tumescence). Polysomnographic assessment of sleep-related erections is useful for differentiating organic from nonorganic erectile dysfunction.

Sleep spindle   Spindle-shaped bursts of 11.5- to 15.0-Hz waves lasting 0.5–1.5 seconds. Generally diffuse, but of highest voltage over the central regions of the head. The amplitude is typically less than 50 µV in the adult. One of the identifying EEG features of non-REM stage II sleep, it may persist into non-REM stages III and IV but is generally not seen in REM sleep.

Sleep stage demarcation   The significant polysomnographic characteristics that distinguish the boundaries of the sleep stages. In certain conditions and with drugs, sleep stage demarcations may be blurred or lost, making it difficult to identify certain stages with certainty or to distinguish the temporal limits of sleep stage lengths.

Sleep stage episode   A sleep stage interval that represents the stage in a non-REM–REM sleep cycle; easiest to comprehend in relation to REM sleep, which is a homogeneous stage (i.e., the fourth REM sleep episode is in the fourth sleep cycle unless a previous REM episode was skipped). If one interval of REM sleep is separated from another by more than 20 minutes, they constitute separate REM sleep episodes (and are in separate sleep cycles); a sleep stage episode may be of any duration.

Sleep stage non-REM   The other major sleep state apart from REM sleep; comprises sleep stages I–IV, which constitute levels in the spectrum of non-REM sleep "depth" or physiologic intensity.

Sleep stage REM   The stage of sleep with highest brain activity, characterized by enhanced brain metabolism and vivid hallucinatory imagery or dreaming. There are spontaneous rapid eye movements, resting muscle activity is suppressed, and awakening threshold to nonsignificant stimuli is high. The EEG is a low-voltage, mixed-frequency, non-alpha record. REM sleep is usually 20–25% of total sleep time. It is also called *paradoxical sleep.*

Sleep stages   Distinctive stages of sleep best demonstrated by polysomnographic recordings of the EEG, EOG, and EMG.

Sleep stage I (non-REM stage I)   A stage of non-REM sleep that occurs at sleep onset or that follows arousal from sleep stages II, III, IV, or REM. It consists of a relatively low-voltage EEG with mixed frequency, mainly theta and alpha activity of less than 50% of the scoring epoch. It contains EEG vertex waves; slow, rolling eye movements; and no sleep spindles, K complexes, or REMs. Stage I normally represents 4–5% of the major sleep episode.

Sleep stage II (non-REM stage II)   A stage of non-REM sleep characterized by the presence of sleep spindles and K complexes present in a relatively low-voltage, mixed-frequency EEG background. High-voltage delta waves may comprise less than 20% of stage II epochs. Stage II usually accounts for 45–55% of the major sleep episode.

Sleep stage III (non-REM stage III)   A stage of non-REM sleep defined by at least 20%, and not more than 50%, of the episode consisting of EEG waves less than 2 Hz and more than 75 µV (high-amplitude delta waves). Stage III is a delta sleep stage. "Deep" non-REM sleep, so-called slow wave sleep, is made up of stages III and IV. Stage III is often combined with stage IV into non-REM sleep stage III/IV because of the lack of documented physiologic differences between the two. Stage III appears usually only in the first third of the sleep episode and typically comprises 4–6% of total sleep time.

Sleep stage IV (non-REM stage IV)   All statements concerning non-REM sleep stage III apply to stage IV except that high-voltage,

EEG slow waves persist during 50% or more of the epoch. Non-REM sleep stage IV usually represents 12–15% of total sleep time. Sleep-walking, night terrors, and confusional arousal episodes generally start in stage IV or during arousals from this stage (see *Sleep stage III*).

Sleep structure   Similar to sleep architecture, sleep structure, in addition to encompassing sleep stages and sleep cycle relationships, assesses the within-stage qualities of the EEG and other physiologic attributes.

Sleep talking   Talking in sleep that usually occurs in the course of transitory arousals from non-REM sleep. It can occur during stage REM sleep, at which time it represents a motor breakthrough of dream speech. Full consciousness is not achieved and no memory of the event remains.

Sleep–wake cycle   The clock-hour relationships of the major sleep and wake episodes in the 24-hour cycle (see *Phase transition; Circadian rhythm*).

Sleep–wake shift (-change, -reversal)   Displacement of sleep, entirely or in part, to a time of customary waking activity, and of waking activity to the time of the major sleep episode. Common in jet lag and shift work.

Sleep–wake transition disorder   A disorder that occurs during the transition from wakefulness to sleep or from one sleep stage to another. A parasomnia, not a dyssomnia.

Slow wave sleep   Sleep characterized by EEG waves of duration slower than 4 Hz. Synonymous with sleep stages III and IV combined (see *Delta sleep stage*).

Snoring   A noise produced primarily with inspiratory respiration during sleep owing to vibration of the soft palate and the pillars of the oropharyngeal inlet. All snorers have incomplete obstruction of the upper airway, and many habitual snorers have complete episodes of upper airway obstruction.

Spindle REM sleep   A condition in which sleep spindles persist atypically during REM sleep, occasionally in the first REM period; seen in chronic insomnia conditions.

Synchronized   A chronobiological term used to indicate that two or more rhythms recur with the same phase relationship. In EEG it is used to indicate increased amplitude—and usually decreased frequency—of the dominant activities.

Theta activity   EEG activity with a frequency of 4.0–7.5 Hz, generally maximal over the central and temporal cortex.

Total recording time   The interval from sleep onset to final awakening. In addition to total sleep time, it is comprised of the time taken up by wake periods and movement time until wake-up (see *Sleep efficiency*).

Total sleep episode   The total time available for sleep during an attempt to sleep. It comprises non-REM and REM sleep as well as wakefulness. Synonymous with (and preferred to) *total sleep period*.

Total sleep time   The amount of actual sleep time in a sleep episode; equal to total sleep episode minus awake time. Total sleep time is the total of all REM and non-REM sleep in a sleep episode.

Tracé alternant   EEG pattern of sleeping newborns, characterized by bursts of slow waves, at times intermixed with sharp waves, and intervening periods of relative quiescence with extreme low-amplitude activity.

Tumescence (penile)   Hardening and expansion of the penis (penile erection). When associated with REM sleep, it is referred to as a *sleep-related erection*.

Twitch (body twitch)   A very small body movement, such as a local foot or finger jerk; not usually associated with arousal.

Vertex sharp transient   Sharp negative potential, maximal at the vertex, occurring spontaneously during sleep or in response to a sensory stimulus during sleep or wakefulness. Amplitude varies but rarely exceeds 250 µV. Use of the term *vertex sharp wave* is discouraged.

Wake time   The total time scored as wakefulness in a polysomnogram occurring between sleep onset and final wake-up.

Waxing and waning   A crescendo-decrescendo pattern of activity, usually EEG activity.

Zeitgeber   German term for an environmental time cue that usually helps entrainment to the 24-hour day, such as sunlight, noise, social interaction, alarm clock.

Index

Acetazolamide, in treatment of obstructive sleep apnea syndrome, 77, 78
Acromegaly and sleep disturbances, 154
Actigraphy, 56
in assessment of insomnia, 90
Adaptive theory of sleep, 8
Adjustment sleep disorder, 188
Advanced sleep phase syndrome, 165–166
Affective disorders and insomnia, 145–146
African sleeping sickness, 157
AIDS and sleep disturbances, 155–156
Akathisia, vs. restless legs syndrome, 121
Alcohol, as cause of sleep disturbances, 148
Aldosterone secretion during sleep, 19
Alimentary system, changes in during sleep, 18
Alzheimer's disease and sleep disturbances, 128–129, 181
treatment of, 144
Amyotrophic lateral sclerosis and sleep disturbances, 130
Angina, nocturnal, and sleep disturbances, 152
Angiotensin-converting enzyme inhibitors and sleep disturbances, 158
Anorectics and sleep disturbances, 158
Anorexia nervosa and sleep disturbances, 147
treatment of, 149
Antidepressants, as cause of sleep disturbances, 148, 159
Antidiuretic hormone secretion during sleep, 19
Antiemetics and sleep disturbances, 158
Antihistamines and sleep disturbances, 158, 159
Apnea. See also Obstructive sleep apnea syndrome
central, and insomnia, 86
and acromegaly, 154
definition of, 69–70

Appetite suppressants and sleep disturbances, 158
Arousal disorders
epidemiology of, 64
genetics of, 67–68
Aspartate and wakefulness, 10
Aspirin and sleep disturbances, 158
Asthma and sleep disturbances, 153–154
in children, 191
Autonomic nervous system, changes in during sleep, 15–17
pupils, 16
sympathetic activity in muscle and skin blood vessels, 16
Autosomal dominant nocturnal frontal lobe epilepsy, 136

Baclofen, in treatment of restless legs syndrome and periodic limb movements in sleep, 125
Bedwetting, persistent, 192
Benign focal epilepsy of childhood, 133–134
Benign temporal delta transients of the elderly, 175
Benzodiazepines, in treatment of insomnia, 91, 93
Beta blockers and sleep disturbances, 158
Biological clock, 161
Blindness, and hypernychthemeral syndrome, 166
Blood pressure, changes in during sleep, 18
Body position, monitoring of during sleep, 27–28
Bootzin's stimulus control technique, for treatment of insomnia, 91, 92
Breathing and sleep disorders. See also Obstructive sleep apnea syndrome
Cheyne-Stokes breathing, 70, 153
hypoventilation, 70
paradoxical breathing, 70
upper airway resistance syndrome, 71

Bromocriptine, in treatment of restless legs syndrome and periodic limb movements in sleep, 124
Bronchodilators and sleep disturbances, 158
Bruxism, 172, 173
Bulimia nervosa and sleep disturbances, 147
treatment of, 149

Capnography, 26–27
Carbamazepine, in treatment of restless legs syndrome and periodic limb movements in sleep, 125
Carbidopa-levodopa, in treatment of restless legs syndrome and periodic limb movements in sleep, 123, 124
Carbon dioxide level, expired, 26–27
Cardiac output, changes in during sleep, 18
Cardiovascular system, changes in during sleep, 18
clinical implications of, 20
Cataplexy, 96, 97
Central sleep apnea–insomnia syndrome, 86
Cheyne-Stokes breathing, 70, 153
Children, sleep disorders in. See Pediatric sleep disorders
Chronic fatigue syndrome and sleep disturbances, 156
Chronic obstructive pulmonary disease and sleep disturbances, 153
Chronobiology, 162–163
Chronopharmacology, 163
Chronotherapy, 163
Circadian rhythms, 4–5, 6, 161–166
in African sleeping sickness, 157
and biological clock, 161
and chronobiology, 162–163
and chronopharmacology, 163
and chronotherapy, 163
disorders of, 163–166. See also Jet lag; Shift work
advanced sleep phase syndrome, 165–166
delayed sleep phase syndrome, 164–165
hypernychthemeral syndrome, 166
in elderly, 176
and suprachiasmatic nucleus, 161–162

Clonazepam
in treatment of restless legs syndrome and periodic limb movements in sleep, 124
in treatment of sleep disturbance in Parkinson's disease, 123
Clonidine, in treatment of restless legs syndrome and periodic limb movements in sleep, 125
Clozapine, in treatment of sleep disturbance in Parkinson's disease, 123
Colic, as cause of sleep disturbances in infants, 191
Confusional arousals, 169
Congestive cardiac failure and sleep disturbances, 153
Continuous positive airway pressure in treatment of obstructive sleep apnea syndrome, 78, 79
adverse effects of, 78, 79
in treatment of sleep disturbances in neurologic disorders, 142

Daytime sleepiness. See Excessive daytime somnolence
Delayed sleep phase syndrome, 164–165
Dementia, and sleep disturbances in the elderly, 179
Dental appliances, in treatment of obstructive sleep apnea syndrome, 78, 79
Depression and insomnia, 145–146
treatment of, 149
Dermatologic disorders and sleep disturbances, 157
Dopamine and wakefulness, 10
Dream anxiety attacks. See Nightmares
Dreams, 6
Duchenne's muscular dystrophy and sleep disturbances, 137
Dyssomnias, 47, 48–49
Dystonia musculorum deformans and sleep, 114

Eating disorders and sleep disturbances, 147
treatment of, 149
Elderly
changes in electroencephalography, sleep architecture, and circadian rhythms in, 4, 175–176
nocturnal confusional episodes in, treatment of, 185–186

physiologic changes in, 176–177, 178
situational stress in, treatment
    of, 185
sleep complaints in, 177–179
sleep cycle changes in, treatment of,
    185
sleep disorders in, 179–186
    assessment of, 182–183
        importance of complete medical
            history, 182
        laboratory assessment, 183
    excessive daytime sleepiness, 180
    frequent awakenings, 181
    insomnia, 180
    medication-induced, treatment
        of, 186
    obstructive sleep apnea syndrome,
        179–180
    periodic limb movements in sleep,
        180–181
    rapid eye movement sleep behav-
        ior disorder, 181
    treatment of, 183–184
        exercise program, 186
        for insomnia, 184
        special pharmacologic consider-
            ations in, 184–185
Electrical status epilepticus, 134
Electro-oculography, 25. See also Scor-
    ing technique
Electrocardiography, 25. See also Scor-
    ing technique
Electroencephalography, 23–24. See
    also Scoring technique
    in elderly, 175
Electromyography, 25. See also Scoring
    technique
Endocrine diseases and sleep distur-
    bances, 155
Energy conservation theory of sleep, 8
Enuresis, primary, 192
Epilepsy and sleep disturbances,
    132–136
    effect of epilepsy on sleep, 136
    effect of sleep on epilepsy, 133–136
        autosomal dominant nocturnal
            frontal lobe epilepsy, 136
        benign focal epilepsy of child-
            hood, 133–134
        electrical status epilepticus, 134
        juvenile myoclonic epilepsy, 134
        nocturnal paroxysmal dystonia,
            134–135
        tonic seizures, 133
Epworth Sleepiness Scale, 31–32

Esophageal motility during sleep, 18
Esophageal pH, monitoring of, 27
Excessive daytime somnolence, 31
    causes of, 51–53
    in the elderly, 180
    epidemiology of, 60–62
    and obstructive sleep apnea syn-
        drome, 75
Excitatory amino acids, and wakeful-
    ness, 10

Fatal familial insomnia. See Insomnia,
    fatal familial
Fiberoptic endoscopy, in assessment of
    obstructive sleep apnea syn-
    drome, 76–77
Fibromyalgia syndrome and sleep dis-
    turbances, 156–157
Food allergy insomnia, 189

GABA, and nonrapid eye movement
    sleep, 13
Gabapentin, in treatment of restless
    legs syndrome and periodic
    limb movements in sleep, 124
Gastric acid secretion, and sleep, 18
Gastroesophageal reflux disease and
    sleep disturbances, 154
    in children, 191
Glutamate, and wakefulness, 10
Gonadotropin secretion during sleep, 19
Growth hormone during sleep, 19

Headache syndromes and sleep distur-
    bances, 138–139
Heart rate, changes in during sleep, 18
Hematologic disorders and sleep dis-
    turbances, 156
Hemorrhagic telangiectasia, heredi-
    tary, and sleep disturbances,
    156
HLA typing, in assessment of nar-
    colepsy, 104
Homeostatic factor, 6–7
Homicide, somnambulistic, 194
Hot flashes, and thermoregulation
    during sleep, 20
Huntington's disease, and sleep,
    113–114
Hypopnea, definition of, 70. See also
    Obstructive sleep apnea
    syndrome
Hypernychthemeral syndrome, 166
Hypersomnia, 51
    in the elderly, 178

Hypersomnia—*continued*
  general medical causes of, 151–152
  idiopathic, 103
    treatment of, 105
  neurologic causes of, 127–128
  and seasonal affective dis-
      order, 145
Hypertension, and obstructive sleep
    apnea syndrome, 153
Hypnic jerks, 171
Hypnotic agents and sleep distur-
    bances, 158
Hypoventilation, 70

Imaging studies, in assessment of
    obstructive sleep apnea syn-
    drome, 76–77
Insomnia, 50, 51, 81–94
  altitude and, 85
  assessment of, 87–90
    actigraphy, 90
    alcohol and drug history, 89
    family history, 89
    laboratory evaluation, 89–90
    physical examination, 89
    sleep diary, 89
    sleep history, 87–88
  causes of, 82–83
    neurologic, 127
  and central sleep apnea, 86
  classification of, 81
  clinical manifestations of, 51, 81–82
  definition of, 81
  in the elderly, 177–178, 180
    treatment of, 184
  epidemiology of, 59–60, 81
  fatal familial, 140
    genetics of, 67
  idiopathic, 84
  and inadequate sleep hygiene, 85
  and insufficient sleep syndrome, 85
  jet lag and, 82
  and long-term health, 82
  medical disorders causing, 86–87
    neurologic, 87
  psychiatric disorders causing, 87,
      145–149. *See also* Psychiatric
      disorders and sleep distur-
      bances
  psychophysiologic, 84
  shift work and, 82–83
  and sleep state misperception, 84
  treatment of, 90–94
    pharmacologic, 91, 92–94
      benzodiazepine hypnotics, 91, 93

nonbenzodiazepine hypnotics,
    91, 93–94
relaxation therapy, 90
sleep hygiene measures, 90, 91
sleep restriction therapy, 92
stimulus control therapy, 91, 92
Insufficient sleep syndrome, 85
Intensive care unit patients and sleep
    disturbances, 155
International Classification of Sleep
    Disorders, 47–50
Intraesophageal pressure monitoring, 27
Ischemic heart disease and sleep dis-
    turbances, 152

Jet lag, 163–164
  and insomnia, 82
  treatment of, 164
Juvenile myoclonic epilepsy, 134

K complex, 39
Kleine-Levin syndrome and sleep dis-
    turbances, 139

Leg cramps, nocturnal, 172
Levodopa, in treatment of sleep distur-
    bance in Parkinson's dis-
    ease, 122
Limb-girdle muscular dystrophy and
    sleep disturbances, 137
Limit-setting sleep disorder, 189
Lithium and sleep disturbances, 159
Lyme disease and sleep distur-
    bances, 156

Maintenance of Wakefulness Test,
    34–35
  in assessment of narcolepsy, 104
  vs. Multiple Sleep Latency Test, 35,
    55–56
Malingering, and sleep-related vio-
    lence, 195
Mean sleep latency, 33
Medications and sleep disturbances,
    113, 148, 149, 158–159
Melatonin
  in prevention of jet lag, 164
  secretion of during sleep, 19, 20
  in treatment of insomnia, 94
  in treatment of shift work sleep dis-
    order, 164
Memory reinforcement and consolida-
    tion of sleep, 8
Menopausal hot flashes, and ther-
    moregulation during sleep, 20

Methylphenidate, in treatment of narcolepsy, 104–105
Migrating motor complex, 18
Modafinil, in treatment of narcolepsy, 104–105
Monitoring and recording, 28. *See also specific monitoring methods*
Monoamine oxidase inhibitors, as cause of sleep disturbances, 148
Movement disorders and sleep disturbances, 108–125
   approach to patient with, 120–122
   Huntington's disease, 113–114
   management of, 122–125
      in Parkinson's disease, 122–123
      in restless legs syndrome and periodic limb movements in sleep, 123–125
   Parkinson's disease. *See* Parkinson's disease
   periodic limb movements. *See* Periodic limb movements in sleep
   physiologic vs. pathologic, 108–110
   progressive supranuclear palsy, 114
   restless legs syndrome. *See* Restless legs syndrome
   torsion dystonia, 114
   Tourette's syndrome, 114–115
Multiple sclerosis and sleep disturbances, 138
Multiple Sleep Latency Test, 31–35
   in assessment of narcolepsy, 104
   indications for, 34
   in obstructive sleep apnea syndrome, 76
   reliability, validity, and limitation of, 33–34
   technique for, 32–33
   vs. Maintenance of Wakefulness Test, 35, 55–56
Multiple system atrophy
   clinical features of, 131
   and sleep disturbances, 129–131
Munchausen syndrome, and sleep-related violence, 195
Myasthenia gravis and sleep disturbances, 137
Myotonic dystrophy and sleep disturbances, 136–137

Narcolepsy, 95–102
   associated features of, 96, 98
   clinical manifestations of, 95–98
      automatic behavior, 96, 98

   cataplexy, 96, 97
   disturbed night sleep, 96, 98
   hypnagogic hallucination, 96, 97–98
   narcoleptic sleep attacks, 96–97
   sleep paralysis, 96, 97
   differential diagnosis of, 98–100
      absence spells, 99
      drop attacks, 100
      idiopathic hypersomnia, 99
      obstructive sleep apnea syndrome, 99
      seizures, 99, 100
      syncope, 100
   epidemiology of, 95
   genetic aspects of, 65–66, 95
   as indication for Multiple Sleep Latency Test, 34
   laboratory assessment of, 103–104
      HLA typing, 104
      Maintenance of Wakefulness Test, 104
      Multiple Sleep Latency Test, 104
      polysomnography, 103–104
   pathogenesis of, 100–102
      genetic and environmental factors, 102
      neurochemical mechanisms, 101–102
      physiologic mechanisms, 100–101
   sleep apnea and, 98, 99
   treatment of, 104–105
      methylphenidate, 104–105
      modafinil, 105
      pemoline, 104–105
   vs. idiopathic hypersomnia, 103
Narcotics and sleep disturbances, 158
Neurodegenerative disorders and sleep disturbances, 128–131
   Alzheimer's disease, 128–129
      treatment of, 144
   amyotrophic lateral sclerosis, 130
   multiple system atrophy, 129–130
   olivopontocerebellar atrophy, 129
Neuroleptics, as cause of sleep disturbances, 148, 159
Neurologic disorders and sleep disturbances, 127–144
   in children, 190–191
   epilepsy. *See* Epilepsy and sleep disturbances
   fatal familial insomnia. *See* Insomnia, fatal familial
   headache syndromes, 138–139
   hypersomnia, 127–128

Neurologic disorders and sleep disturbances—*continued*
idiopathic recurrent stupor, 139–140
insomnia, 127
Kleine-Levin syndrome, 139
laboratory investigations of, 140–141
management of, 141–144
  nasal continuous positive airway pressure, 142
  negative-pressure or positive-pressure ventilation, 142–143
  objective of, 141–142
  supplemental oxygen therapy, 143
  surgery, 143–144
multiple sclerosis, 138
neurodegenerative disorders. *See* Neurodegenerative disorders and sleep disturbances
neuromuscular disorders, 136–137
poliomyelitis and postpolio syndrome, 137
spinal cord diseases, 137–138
stroke, 132
traumatic brain injuries, 139
Neuromuscular disorders and sleep disturbances, 136–137
Newborns
scoring techniques for, 42, 44–45
  for electroencephalogram, 42, 45
  for electromyogram, 44, 45
  for eye movements, 44, 45
  for respiration, 42, 45
sleep patterns in, 4
Night terrors. *See* Sleep terrors
Nightmares, 169–170
epidemiology of, 64
Nocturnal eating (drinking) syndrome, 189
Nocturnal paroxysmal dystonia, 134–135
Nonbenzodiazepines, in treatment of insomnia, 91, 93–94
Nonrapid eye movement sleep, 1–3
active vs. passive cycling of, 10–11
behavioral criteria for, 2
cardiovascular changes during, 18
dreams during, 6
GABA and, 13
humoral sleep factors and, 12–13
hypnogenic neurons responsible for, 11
motor system changes during, 107–108

nucleus of the tractus solitarius and, 12
physiologic changes during, 15–17
physiologic criteria for, 2, 3
respiration and, 17
rhythms of, and slow cortical oscillations, 12–13
scoring technique for, 37–39
serotonin and, 13
Non–24-hour sleep–wake disorder, 166
Nucleus of the tractus solitarius, and nonrapid eye movement sleep, 12

Obesity-hypoventilation syndrome, 74
Obsessive-compulsive disorder and sleep disturbances, 146–147
treatment of, 149
Obstructive sleep apnea syndrome, 69–80, 189–190. *See also* Breathing and sleep disorders
apnea, definition of, 69–70
and chronic obstructive pulmonary disease (overlap syndrome), 153
consequences of, 71–72
in the elderly, 179–180
epidemiology of, 62–63, 71
genetic studies in, 68
and hypertension, 153
hypopnea, definition of, 70
imaging studies, 76–77
laboratory assessment of, 75–77
  Multiple Sleep Latency Test, 76
  polysomnography, 75–76
management of, 77–80
  general measures, 77–78
  mechanical devices, 78, 79
  pharmacologic, 78
  surgical, 78–80
and narcolepsy, 98, 99
and obesity-hypoventilation syndrome (pickwickian syndrome), 74
pathogenesis of, 73–74
respiratory disturbance index, 70
risk factors for, 71, 72
physical findings in, 75
pulmonary function tests, 77
and stroke, 132
symptoms and signs of, 74–75
and violent behavior, 194
Olivopontocerebellar atrophy and sleep disturbances, 129

Ondine's curse, 132
Opiates, in treatment of restless legs syndrome and periodic limb movements in sleep, 124
Overlap syndrome, 153
Oxygen saturation, 26
Oxygen therapy, supplemental, in treatment of sleep disturbances in neurologic disorders, 143

Pain and sleep disturbances, 157–158
Panic disorder and sleep disturbances, 146
    treatment of, 149
Paradoxical breathing, 70
Parasomnias, 47, 48–49, 167–173. See also Nightmares; Sleep terrors; Sleep talking; Sleepwalking
    assessment and treatment of, 173
    benign neonatal sleep myoclonus, 172–173
    bruxism, 172, 173
    classification of, 167
    confusional arousals, 169
    epidemiology of, 63–64
    genetic studies of, 67–68
    hypnic jerks, 171
    isolated sleep paralysis, 171
    nocturnal leg cramps, 172
    rapid eye movement sleep behavior disorder, 68, 170
    rhythmic movement disorder, 171–172
Parkinson's disease
    clinical features of, 110, 111
    and sleep disturbance, 111–113, 181
        and associated conditions, 113
        effect of antiparkinsonian medications on sleep, 113
        effect of disease on sleep, 111–112
        effect of sleep on disease, 112–113
        management of, 122–123
Paroxysmal nocturnal hemoglobinuria and sleep disturbances, 156
Pavor nocturnus. See Sleep terrors
Pediatric sleep disorders, 187–192
    adjustment sleep disorder, 188
    caused by general medical disorders, 191
    caused by neurologic disorders, 190–191
    caused by psychiatric disorders, 191–192
    food allergy insomnia, 189

limit-setting sleep disorder, 189
    nocturnal eating (drinking) syndrome, 189
    obstructive sleep apnea syndrome, 189–190
    primary enuresis, 192
    sleep-onset association disorder, 188–189
Pemoline, in treatment of narcolepsy, 104–105
Peptic ulcer disease and sleep disturbances, 154
Pergolide, in treatment of restless legs syndrome and periodic limb movements in sleep, 124
Periodic limb movement disorder, 116
Periodic limb movements in sleep, 115–117
    and associated conditions, 116–117
    diagnosis of, 115
    in the elderly, 180–181
    prevalence of, 117
Periodic limb movements in wakefulness, 115
Pickwickian syndrome, 74
Piezoelectric strain gauges, 26
Poliomyelitis and postpolio syndrome, sleep disturbances in, 137
Polyneuropathies and sleep disturbances, 137
Polysomnography, 21–23. See also Scoring technique
    indications for, 28–29
    instructions for physiologic calibrations, 22
    in obstructive sleep apnea syndrome, 75–76
    patient preparation and laboratory environment, 21–22
    portable, 29–30
    technical considerations for, 22–23
    video, 56
Post-traumatic stress disorder and sleep disturbances, 147
    treatment of, 149
Pramipexole, in treatment of restless legs syndrome and periodic limb movements in sleep, 124
Progressive supranuclear palsy, and sleep, 114
Prolactin secretion during sleep, 19
Propranolol, in treatment of restless legs syndrome and periodic limb movements in sleep, 125

Protriptyline, in treatment of obstructive sleep apnea syndrome, 77, 78
Pruritus and sleep disturbances, 157
Psychiatric disorders and sleep disturbances, 145–149
    anxiety disorders, 146–147, 149
    assessment and treatment of, 148–149
    in children, 191–192
    depression, 145–146, 149
    eating disorders, 147, 149
    and medications, 148, 149
    schizophrenia, 147, 149
Psychogenic dissociative state, 195
Pulmonary function tests, in assessment of obstructive sleep apnea syndrome, 77
Pupils, changes in during sleep, 16

Rapid eye movement sleep behavior disorder, 68, 170
    in the elderly, 181
    and violent behavior, 194
Rapid eye movement sleep
    active vs. passive cycling of, 10–11
    behavioral criteria for, 2
    cardiovascular changes during, 18
    dreams during, 6
    motor system changes during, 107–108
    muscle hypotonia or atonia in, 14
    phasic stage of, 3
    physiologic changes during, 15–17
    physiologic criteria for, 2,3–4
    pons and, 13
    REM-on and REM-off cells in, 13–14
    respiration and, 17
    scoring technique for, 38, 40
    tonic stage of, characteristics of, 3
Rechtschaffen and Kales' technique for scoring. See Scoring technique
Reflux esophagitis and sleep disturbances, 154
Renal failure, chronic, and sleep disturbances, 154–155
Respiration during sleep, 17
    clinical implications of, 20
    monitoring of, 26
    scoring technique for, 40–41
Respiratory disturbance index, 70
Restless legs syndrome, 117–120
    causes of, 119–120
    course of, 119

diagnosis of, 117, 118
differential diagnosis of, 120–121
    akathisia, 121
genetic studies of, 66–67
neurologic examination of, 118–119
onset of, 119
and periodic limb movements in sleep, 118
physiologic mechanism of, 120
sensory manifestations of, 117
uremic, 154–155
Restorative theory of sleep, 7
Ritalin, in treatment of narcolepsy, 104–105

Schizophrenia and sleep disturbances, 147
    treatment of, 149
Scoring technique, 37–45
    for arousals, 41–42
    for movement time, body movements, and movement arousal, 40
    in newborns. See Newborns, scoring techniques for
    for nonrapid eye movement sleep
        stage I, 37–39
        stage II, 38, 39
        stage III, 38, 39
        stage IV, 38, 39
    of periodic limb movements in sleep, 41
    for rapid eye movement sleep, 38, 40
    of respiratory events, 40–41
    sample polysomnographic report, 43–44
    for wakefulness, 37, 38
Seasonal affective disorder and hypersomnolence, 145
Seizures. See also Epilepsy and sleep disturbances
    frontal lobe, 134–135
    nonepileptic, 135
    sleep-related, 195–196
    tonic, 133
Serotonin secretion during sleep, 13, 19
Sexual function during sleep, 19
    in elderly, 177
Shift work, 164
    and insomnia, 82–83
Shy-Drager syndrome and sleep disturbances, 129–130
Sickle cell anemia and sleep disturbances, 156

Sleep. *See also* Sleep disorders; *other Sleep entries*
  alimentary changes during, 18
  behavioral criteria for, 1, 2
  cardiovascular system and, 18
  common complaints about, 50
  deprivation and sleepiness, 7
  and dreams, 6
  endocrine function and, 19
  function of, 7–8
  habits of, 5
  mechanisms of, 9–14. *See also* Non-rapid eye movement sleep; Rapid eye movement sleep; Wakefulness
    active vs. passive, 10–11
  motor systems and, 107–108
  movement disorders and. *See* Movement disorders and sleep disturbances
  and neurologic disorders. *See* Neurologic disorders and sleep disturbances
  patterns of
    in newborns, 4
    in old age, 4
  physiologic changes in, 15–20
    alimentary, 18
    in autonomic nervous system. *See* Autonomic nervous system, changes in during sleep
    cardiovascular, 18
    clinical implications of, 20
    endocrine, 19
    respiratory, 17
    sexual, 19
    in somatic central nervous system, 15
    thermoregulatory, 19–20
  physiologic criteria for, 1, 2
  requirements for, 5
  respiration and, 17
  sexual function during, 19
  stages of, 1–3. *See also* Nonrapid eye movement sleep; Rapid eye movement sleep
  vs. coma, 9
Sleep apnea. *See* Obstructive sleep apnea syndrome
Sleep disorders
  approach to patients with, 50–57
    clinical evaluation, 53–55
      family history for, 55
      physical examination for, 55
      sleep log for, 55
    laboratory assessment, 55–57. *See also* Maintenance of Wakefulness Test; Multiple Sleep Latency Test
      actigraphy, 56
      video-polysomnography, 56
  associated with medical/psychiatric disorders, 48
  classification of, 47–50
  dyssomnias, 47, 48–49
  epidemiology of, 59–64
  genetics of, 65–68
  hypersomnia, 51
  insomnia. *See* Insomnia
  parasomnias. *See* Parasomnias
  proposed, 48–49
Sleep hygiene
  inadequate, 85
  measures for treatment of insomnia, 90, 91
Sleeping pills and sleep disturbances, 158
Sleep logs, 55
  for assessment of insomnia, 89
Sleep-onset association disorder, 188–189
Sleep paralysis
  epidemiology of, 64
  genetics of, 68
  isolated, 171
  in narcolepsy, 96, 97
Sleep spindles, 39
Sleep state misperception, 84
"Sleep starts," 171
Sleep talking, 172
  epidemiology of, 64
  genetics of, 67–68
Sleep terrors, 168–169
  epidemiology of, 64
  genetics of, 67–68
Sleepwalking, 167–168
  genetics of, 67–68
Slow wave sleep, 39
Snoring
  in the elderly, 179, 180
  epidemiology of, 62
  monitoring of, 27
  and obstructive sleep apnea syndrome, 180
  and stroke, 132
Spinal cord diseases and sleep disturbances, 137–138
Stanford Sleepiness Scale, 31, 32
Status dissociatus, 195
Status epilepticus, electrical, 134

Stroke and sleep disturbances, 132
Suprachiasmatic nucleus, 161–162
"Sundowning" in Alzheimer's disease, 129
Synaptic and neuronal network maintenance theory of sleep, 8

Teenagers, sleep and, 53
Temazepam, in treatment of restless legs syndrome and periodic limb movements in sleep, 124
Testosterone secretion during sleep, 19
Theophylline and sleep disturbances, 158
Thermistor, 26
Thermocouple device, 26
Thermoregulation
  changes in during sleep, 19–20
  and menopausal hot flashes, 20
  and theory of sleep, 8
Thyroid-stimulating hormone secretion during sleep, 19
Tongue-retaining device, in treatment of obstructive sleep apnea syndrome, 78, 79
Tonic seizures, 133
Torsion dystonia, and sleep, 114
Tourette's syndrome, and sleep, 114–115
Tramadol, in treatment of restless legs syndrome and periodic limb movements in sleep, 124
Traumatic brain injuries and sleep disturbances, 139
Tricyclic antidepressants, as cause of sleep disturbances, 148, 159

Trypanosomiasis, 157

Upper airway resistance syndrome, 71
Uvulopalatopharyngoplasty, in treatment of obstructive sleep apnea syndrome, 78–80

Ventilation, negative-pressure or positive-pressure, in treatment of sleep disturbances in neurologic disorders, 142–143
Video monitoring during sleep, 27
Violence, sleep-related, 193–197
  etiology of, 193–194
  evaluation of patients with, 196
  forensic implications of, 197
  and malingering and Munchausen syndrome, 195
  management of patients with, 196
  and psychogenic dissociate state, 195
  and sleep seizures, 195
  and status dissociatus, 195
Visual Analog Scale of Alertness and Well-Being, 31

Wakefulness
  mechanisms of, 9–10
    cholinergic neurons and, 10
    dopamine and, 10
    glutamate and aspartate and, 10
  physiologic changes during, 16
  respiration and, 17
Wisconsin Sleep Cohort Study, 63

Zolpidem, 91, in treatment of insomnia, 93